Paediatrics

A Clinical Handbook

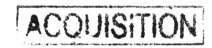

The Paediatrics Ward

At the door to every paediatrics ward
there is a box.
This is where you leave your ego.
Uncloak your shoulders
from your adult cynicism.
See the world through a child's eyes.

Remember, there is no room for your pride here,
it is too full of all the possibilities
of what these children may one day be.
Remind yourself why you're here;
to advocate, to educate,
to give these children a safe space.

And for those children
To whom life has already been cruel,
and those destined to join Peter Pan,
Already on their way
Towards the second star on the right,
And might not make it to the morning

Give them everything you can,
Even if all you have is kindness.
This is a place for healing,
Laughing, growing,
Sometimes grieving,
But above all hope.

So leave your cloak at the door,
Don't your shoulders feel better already?
Welcome, take a seat, let's begin.

Anouska Lerner

Paediatrics

A Clinical Handbook

Joe Esland
Specialty Trainee in Trauma and Orthopaedic Surgery, Edinburgh

Anouska Lerner
Specialty Trainee in Paediatrics, London

Arif Khan
Consultant Paediatric Neurologist and Medical Director,
Neuropedia Children's Neuroscience Center, Dubai, UAE

Scion

Scion Publishing Limited

The Old Hayloft, Vantage Business Park, Bloxham Road, Banbury OX16 9UX, UK
www.scionpublishing.com

Important Note from the Publisher

The information contained within this book was obtained by Scion Publishing Ltd from sources believed by us to be reliable. However, while every effort has been made to ensure its accuracy, no responsibility for loss or injury whatsoever occasioned to any person acting or refraining from action as a result of information contained herein can be accepted by the authors or publishers.

Readers are reminded that medicine is a constantly evolving science and while the authors and publishers have ensured that all dosages, applications and practices are based on current indications, there may be specific practices which differ between communities. You should always follow the guidelines laid down by the manufacturers of specific products and the relevant authorities in the country in which you are practising.

Although every effort has been made to ensure that all owners of copyright material have been acknowledged in this publication, we would be pleased to acknowledge in subsequent reprints or editions any omissions brought to our attention.

Registered names, trademarks, etc. used in this book, even when not marked as such, are not to be considered unprotected by law.

Our medical textbooks are assessed and reviewed by the following medical students:

Nora Aljamil	Umar Dinah	Marco Narajas
Adam Arshad	Keziah Element	Toby Nicholls
Tanith Bain	Sophie Gunter	Simran Piya
Susan Baird	Laura Hartley	Ross Porter
Nabeela Bhaloo	Zoe Johnson	Macauley Shaw
Amy Campbell	Victoria Kinkaid	Jay Singh
Thomas Charles	Dylan McClurg	Paris Tatt-Smith
Jason Cheong Kah Chun	Connor McKee	Charlotte Thompson
Yasmine Cherfi	Kate McMurrugh	Jack Whiting
Amaan Din	Jonathan Mok	

We are grateful for their essential feedback. If you would like to apply to be a student reviewer, please contact **simon.watkins@scionpublishing.com** in the first instance.

Typeset by Medlar Publishing Solutions Pvt Ltd, India
Printed in the UK
Last digit is the print number: 10 9 8 7 6 5 4 3 2 1

Contents

Contents

> **Self-assessment questions**
> Self-assessment questions can be found by clicking on the 'Resources' tab at www.scionpublishing.com/Paediatrics. A selection of short answer questions and single best answer (SBA) questions can be found there, together with their answers. These are the style of questions most commonly used across medical schools in the UK.

Preface

Paediatrics is a vast specialty; it encompasses all body systems, as well as the breadth of medical and surgical conditions that affect them. It is made more challenging because childhood anatomy and physiology differs from that of adults, and then changes as children develop. This means that you cannot simply 'translate' the signs and symptoms of adult disease into childhood – you must learn paediatrics from first principles.

It is also important to recognise that paediatrics introduces a number of unique challenges in the clinical environment. Examples might include recognising the features of child abuse, dealing with anxious parents or assessing capacity to consent; the list is long and you will definitely encounter these situations as you progress through your training.

Paediatrics: a clinical handbook was written after the authors recognised the need for a textbook that was an effective balance between an overly concise text and an excessively detailed one. With a focus on providing clear, clinically relevant content, presented in a structure that helps to promote a deep understanding of the information from first principles, it is hoped that this book will act as a valuable resource in undergraduate clinical training and for new doctors on the ward.

Joe Esland
Anouska Lerner
Arif Khan

Acknowledgements

Joe:

I would like to thank my fiancée, Rachel, without whose ongoing support and encouragement the book would not have been completed. Additionally, I'd like to thank all of the hard-working, inspiring and often undervalued medical students with whom I've worked, who frequently remind me of the main purpose for writing this book.

Anouska:

There are many people without whom this project would not have been completed. Firstly, thank you to my wonderful parents Richard and Pip, for your enduring love and support. For always telling me you believed in me and therefore allowing me to believe in myself.

To my sister Debbie, for being my biggest cheerleader and always encouraging me to follow the path I wanted, and not the one most travelled.

To my medical sister Emily, for being such an amazing support from day one of medical school, and still being my sounding post all these years later.

To Joe Esland, for his encouragement and vision; thank you for the opportunity that started in the midst of a busy A&E job.

To Viraf for always being so wonderful, patient and kind. Your endless love, care and encouragement are what allow me to continue caring for and encouraging other people, both at work and outside it.

To all the wonderful consultants, registrars, peers and colleagues that have inspired me in my career so far, not least Graham Derrick at Great Ormond Street Hospital, all the amazing consultants at Evelina Children's Hospital and my wonderful mentor Mojgan Ezzati at University Hospital Lewisham.

Lastly, to all the children I have cared for and will care for in the future, thank you for always giving me hope, and always making me smile.

Arif:

I'm eternally grateful to my parents, who taught me discipline, manners, respect and so much more that has helped me succeed in life. As I was going through a major shift with my career and personal circumstances, I received unending moral support and encouragement from my lovely wife Arva. I would like to thank her for always being the person I could turn to during moments of despair and darkness.

Having an idea and turning it into a book is as hard as it sounds. I especially want to thank Joe, a young doctor, without whose energy, motivation and discipline this book would never have seen the light of day.

Abbreviations

ACE	angiotensin-converting enzyme	ED	Emergency Department
ADHD	attention deficit hyperactivity disorder	ENT	ear, nose and throat
		ESR	erythrocyte sedimentation rate
AED	anti-epileptic drug	ETN	erythema toxicum neonatorum
AIS	adolescent idiopathic scoliosis	FB	foreign body
ALP	alkaline phosphatase	FBC	full blood count
ASD	atrial septal defect / autistic spectrum disorder	FII	fabricated or induced illness
		FTT	failure to thrive
ASOT	antistreptolysin O titre	GCS	Glasgow Coma Scale
AVSD	atrioventricular septal defect	GH	growth hormone
AXR	abdominal X-ray	GI	gastrointestinal
BBB	blood–brain barrier	GMC	General Medical Council
BHS	breath-holding spell	GMFCS	Gross Motor Function Classification System
CA	Cobb angle		
CD	coeliac disease	GN	glomerulonephritis
CHD	congenital heart disease	GORD	gastro-oesophageal reflux disease
CHF	congestive heart failure	HIV	human immunodeficiency virus
CKD	chronic kidney disease	HLHS	hypoplastic left heart syndrome
CMPI	cow's milk protein intolerance	HPC	history of presenting complaint
CMV	cytomegalovirus	HPGA	hypothalamic–pituitary–gonadal axis
CNS	central nervous system		
CP	cerebral palsy	HPV	human papillomavirus
CPAP	continuous positive airway pressure	HR	heart rate
CRP	C-reactive protein	HSP	Henoch–Schönlein purpura
CRT	capillary refill time	HSV	herpes simplex virus
CSF	cerebrospinal fluid	HTN	hypertension
CT	computerized tomography	HUS	haemolytic uraemic syndrome
CXR	chest X-ray	IBD	inflammatory bowel disease
DANISH	Dysdiadochokinesia, Ataxia, Nystagmus, Intention tremor, Speech, Hypotonia	IBS	irritable bowel syndrome
		ICP	intracranial pressure
		IE	infective endocarditis
DH	dermatitis herpetiformis; drug history	ILAE	International League Against Epilepsy
DM	diabetes mellitus	ITP	idiopathic thrombocytopenic purpura
DMARD	disease-modifying antirheumatic drug		
		IUGR	intrauterine growth restriction
DMD	Duchenne muscular dystrophy	IV	intravenous
EBV	Epstein–Barr virus	IVH	intraventricular haemorrhage

JIA	juvenile idiopathic arthritis	ROM	range of movement
KD	Kawasaki disease	ROP	retinopathy of prematurity
LBW	low birthweight	RR	respiratory rate
LDH	lactate dehydrogenase	RSV	respiratory syncytial virus
LFT	liver function test	RV	right ventricle
LLQ	left lower quadrant	RVH	right ventricular hypertrophy
LP	lumbar puncture	SA	septic arthritis
LRTI	lower respiratory tract infection	SALT	speech and language therapist
MA	mesenteric adenitis	SCBU	special care baby unit
MCUG	micturating cystourogram	SCD	sickle cell disease
MCV	mean cell volume	SCFE	slipped capital femoral epiphysis
MRI	magnetic resonance imaging	SH	social history
NAHI	non-accidental head injury	SIADH	syndrome of inappropriate antidiuretic hormone
NAI	non-accidental injury		
NBM	nil by mouth	SIRS	systemic inflammatory response syndrome
NEC	necrotizing enterocolitis		
NF	neurofibromatosis	SLE	systemic lupus erythematosus
NG	nasogastric	SVC	superior vena cava
NICU	neonatal intensive care unit	SVT	supraventricular tachycardia
NSAID	non-steroidal anti-inflammatory drug	T	temperature
		TB	tuberculosis
NTD	neural tube defect	TdP	torsades de pointes
OCD	obsessive–compulsive disorder	TFT	thyroid function test
ORS	oral rehydration salts	TGA	transposition of the great arteries
PDA	patent ductus arteriosus	TMJ	temporomandibular joint
PE	pulmonary embolism	TOF	tetralogy of Fallot
PEFR	peak expiratory flow rate	TPN	total parenteral nutrition
PMH	past medical history	U&Es	urea and electrolytes
PNES	psychogenic non-epileptic seizure	UC	ulcerative colitis
PR	per rectum	UMN	upper motor neurone
PROM	premature rupture of membranes	URTI	upper respiratory tract infection
PSGN	post-streptococcal glomerulonephritis	USS	ultrasound
		UTI	urinary tract infection
PUO	pyrexia of unknown origin	VLBW	very low birthweight
PVL	periventricular leukomalacia	VP	ventriculoperitoneal
PVR	pulmonary vascular resistance	VSD	ventricular septal defect
RBBB	right bundle branch block	VUR	vesicoureteric reflux
RDS	respiratory distress syndrome	VZV	varicella zoster virus
RLQ	right lower quadrant	WPW	Wolff–Parkinson–White syndrome

Outline of the book

Chapters 1 to *4* provide the information needed to ensure a firm grounding in the core theory of childhood physiology, development and clinical assessment. This is needed in order to appreciate the unique conditions from which children suffer or, where a disease is seen across both childhood and adulthood, how and why the symptoms and signs in children may differ.

Chapter 5 is set aside to discuss child abuse, which should be meaningfully understood by all doctors. Thereafter, chapters are divided by organ system, within which the most important paediatric conditions are described.

Each section follows a similar structure:

- **Pathophysiology:** this describes the pertinent information needed to understand the condition.
- **Epidemiology and risk factors:** this section sets out the prevalence and incidence, and describes relevant risk factors.
- **Symptoms and signs:** these are described in a standardized way, which we hope provides a consistent approach that medical students can use when assessing patients.
- **Diagnosis and investigations:** investigations are listed in the order that they would occur in the clinical environment, beginning with the bedside and non-invasive tests, through blood tests, imaging and invasive diagnostic procedures. A differential diagnosis list is also provided, although this can only really be meaningfully developed experientially, by spending time on placement.
- **Management:** finally, management steps are described, again with a focus on how they would occur in the clinical environment.

Throughout this text a series of features have been utilized to highlight information, including:

Clinical pharmacology	Important aspects of paediatric prescribing are highlighted here
OSCE tips	Utilized throughout this book, these are intended to highlight knowledge commonly assessed in medical school examinations, or clinical skills of particularly high utility
Rapid diagnosis	Guides you quickly to the important diagnostic information
Red Flags boxes	Warns you about life-threatening scenarios

Finally, *Appendix A* provides a list of system-specific symptoms to help guide your history taking.

Chapter 1

History taking and examination

The paediatric history

As the adage goes, '*listen to your patient, they are telling you the diagnosis*'. In this chapter, the foundations of the paediatric history are laid out with particular **focus on the nuances that differentiate it** from the adult counterpart.

It is assumed that the reader already has a good grasp of the general medical history, as well as the system-specific symptoms, before commencing their paediatric training. With this in mind, the below includes only questions that are asked **in addition** to those that one would usually ask in a normal adult history. Where a whole section of the history is new (see *Table 1.1*), all new questions are listed.

Introduction

It is important to remember to introduce yourself to both the child and the people with them, usually addressing the child first. This early interaction is often a useful indicator of how able the child will be to provide a history. In reality, the history is often taken both from the child, **as well as the collateral history**.

Nomenclature of child ages
Newborn – immediately after birth
Neonate – first 28 days of life
Infant – 28 days to 1 year
Child – 1–18 years

- Who is with the child? Do not assume that it is their mother and/or father.
- What is the age of the child?

History of presenting complaint

- As in adults. Allow the patient or their carer to tell you the presenting symptoms, and explore the characteristics and qualities of these **fully before moving on**.
- Next, screen for the other symptoms from the likely causal body system.
- See *Appendix A* for a full list of the system-specific symptoms that should be asked.

Systems review

- As in adults, ask a few questions to screen for pathology of **all the other systems**.
  - This is of particular importance in infants and young children who *commonly present with vague, non-specific symptoms*.
- Plus:
  - **Dermatology:**
    - Has the child developed any new rashes? Many childhood diseases are associated with a rash.
  - **Neurology:**
    - Is the child drowsy?
    - Any neck stiffness?

Table 1.1: Overall structure of the paediatric history
Introduction
Presenting complaint
History of presenting complaint
Systems review, to include: • dermatology • neurology • dehydration
'BiFID' – Birth, Feeding, Immunizations and Development
Past medical / surgical history
Drug history
Family history
Social history

- – Photophobia / phonophobia? Especially in a febrile child, a high index of suspicion for meningitis is always needed – it is therefore good practice to ask about these as a matter of routine.
- Features of **dehydration:**
  - – Is the child still producing **wet nappies**?
  - – Are they thirsty?
  - – Do they produce **tears when they cry**?

'BiFID' – birth, feeding, immunizations and development

Birth – a good birth history is essential
- Antenatal: any problems during the pregnancy?
- Antepartum: any problems with the labour? How were they delivered? How many weeks' gestation (term = 37–42 weeks)? How much did they weigh?
- Postpartum: did they require any neonatal special care? If so, what?

Feeding – particularly if the patient is an infant, take time to find out exactly how much they've been taking
- What do they eat (e.g. breast milk, formula milk, solids)?
- How much do they eat normally (normal is ≤150ml/kg)? And since they've been unwell?
- Still producing wet and/or dirty nappies?

BiFID

Immunizations – important when considering possible aetiologies
- 'Are they fully up to date?' is usually adequate. See box below and *Table 3.1*.

Development – this is not a full developmental assessment (see *Chapter 2*), it is just for an overview. Ask, when did the child first:
- smile? (~6 weeks)
- sit up on their own? (6–8 months)
- walk? (~12 months)
- say their first words *with meaning*? (~12 months)

Past medical / surgical, drug and family history

- As for adults.
- If a patient has a previous medical condition it is useful to ask:
  - When was it diagnosed?
  - What treatment have they received?
  - Who are they under the care of (name of consultant) and at which hospital?
  - When is their next clinic appointment or have they been discharged from follow-up?

UK immunization schedule Autumn 2018 (see also *Table 3.1*)	
2 months	DTaP/IPV/Hib/HepB; PCV; MenB; Rotavirus
3 months	DTaP/IPV/Hib/HepB; Rotavirus
4 months	DTaP/IPV/Hib/HepB; PCV;`MenB
12 months	Hib/MenC; PCV; MMR, MenB
Annually from 2–8 years	Live influenza vaccine
3 years 4 months	DTap/IPV; MMR
Females aged 12	HPV
14 years	Td/IPV; MenACWY

- Drug history – ensure that you remember to ask about allergy status and **when and what the reaction was**.
- Family history – some people find it useful to draw a **family pedigree chart**.

Social history

- Who do they live with at home? Siblings?
  - **Is there currently, or has there ever been, any social care involvement with this child or their siblings?** This is an important question that should always be asked irrespective of the preconceptions you may have about the parents. Requiring a degree of sensitivity to ask, it is useful to fire a 'warning shot', such as "this is a standard question we ask everyone".
- Are they at school?
- Are there any smokers in the home?

Ideas, concerns and expectations (ICE)

This aspect of the paediatric history is very important; it is essential to recognize that having an unwell child is a highly anxious time for the parents, who will often worry that their child has a serious illness. **Addressing these ideas and concerns specifically** will improve your rapport with the parents and increase their satisfaction with the consultation.

You may find the following questions useful:

- Do you have any specific concerns about what the problem might be?
- Are there any specific conditions that you've heard about and that are worrying you?
- Were there any tests or treatments that you were expecting we would provide for your child today?

1.2 The paediatric examination

1.2.1 Hydration status

Assessment of hydration status is a **core part** of the examination of children. Associated with some obvious aetiologies, such as illnesses causing diarrhoea and vomiting, many other non-specific illnesses can cause a child to stop feeding optimally. When protracted, this can lead to dehydration due to inadequate input and it is therefore not uncommonly seen in unwell children.

Clinical features

The clinical features of dehydration (see *Fig. 1.1*) can be categorized into two broad groups: initially, features of depletion of the **interstitial** fluid volume and, later, depletion of the **intravascular** fluid volume.

Clinical features of dehydration	
Interstitial volume depletion	***Intravascular volume depletion***
<ul><li>Dry mucous membranes</li><li>Dry tongue</li><li>Sunken anterior fontanelle</li><li>Sunken eyes and ↓ tears</li><li>Reduced skin turgor (best assessed by pinching the skin of the abdomen or thigh)</li></ul>	<ul><li>Altered consciousness / responsiveness (→ cerebral hypoperfusion)</li><li>Reduced urine output (→ manifesting as increased number of dry nappies)</li><li>Tachypnoea</li><li>Tachycardia ± weak pulse pressure</li><li>↑ capillary refill time</li><li>Falling blood pressure</li></ul>

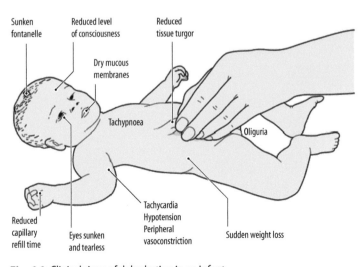

Fig. 1.1: Clinical signs of dehydration in an infant.

Assessing degree of dehydration

When assessing dehydration, it is important to assess the ***degree of severity***. Clinical features are used to **determine if it is mild**, **moderate or severe**: each of these degrees represents the approximate ***percentage loss of body weight as water*** (see *Table 1.2*). This then allows you to prescribe the correct volume of fluid that will need replacing.

Table 1.2: Degree of dehydration			
Degree of severity	**Mild**	**Moderate**	**Severe**
Body weight lost as water	<5%	5–10%	>10%
Clinical features	• Few signs • ± dry mucous membranes	• Dry mucous membranes • Dry tongue • Sunken fontanelle • Reduced skin turgor	• As before plus: • Reduced urine output • Sunken eyes* • Tachycardia* • Tachypnoea* • Altered consciousness or responsiveness*

Progression to shock and parental recognition of Red Flags

When you are sending a child home who is **at risk** of progression to hypovolaemic shock, it is important that you make **parents aware** of the clinical features that indicate that the child is moving towards that point. NICE (2009, CG84) recommends telling parents about the features marked with an asterisk (*) in *Table 1.2*. The clinical features of a child in hypovolaemic shock are, in addition to the above:

- Pale / mottled skin
- Cool extremities
- Weak peripheral pulses
- ↑ capillary refill time
- Hypotension.

1.2.2 General examination

In this section, we are referring to the **observational** assessment you will perform irrespective of the system that is being examined primarily.

- Always begin with observing the child playing in the **waiting room** – this is a good general indicator of growth / nutrition, hygiene and illness severity.
- **Assess growth formally** – height (>2 y/o) or length (<2 y/o), weight and head circumference (in infants). To do the latter, measure the largest circumference of the head (which is between the brow and the occiput) three times, and **take the largest** measurement.
- Hands – cyanosis, clubbing and capillary refill time – either at the nail bed or press over the sternum.

- Head – **palpate the fontanelle** in infants.
- Face – Look for **dysmorphic features**, suggestive of chromosomal or syndromic conditions.
- Skin – it is useful in children to **expose the skin** and look for new rashes.

1.2.3 Respiratory

Inspection

- Count the respiratory rate (see *Table 1.3*)

Table 1.3: Respiratory rate based on a child's age				
Age (years)	0–1	1–5	6–12	>12
Respiratory rate	25–40	20–30	20–25	15–20

- Drooling – a sign of a partially obstructed airway.
- Chest:
  - Inspect for **s**kin changes, **s**cars, **s**welling or a**s**ymmetry
  - Listen for any additional airway sounds such as:
    - **grunting:** a sign of serious illness, produced by exhaling against a partially closed glottis. Localizes pathology to the lower respiratory tract.
    - **stridor:** a harsh breathing sound due to breathing through narrowed upper airway, so localizing pathology to this part of the tract. It may be both inspiratory and expiratory. In a relaxed child it may not be audible but will manifest if the child becomes distressed. Do not examine the child's mouth or throat if you hear this sound, as it may cause laryngospasm.
    - **wheeze:** a high-pitched musical, whistling noise usually heard during expiration. Polyphonic wheeze usually represents asthma, whilst a monophonic wheeze (same pitched wheeze with each breath and the same across the chest) indicates a fixed narrowing – consider an inhaled foreign body.
- Signs of acute respiratory distress:
  - nasal flaring
  - tracheal tug and intercostal recession
  - use of accessory muscles
  - Chronic changes:
    - barrel chest
    - Harrison's sulcus (see *Fig. 1.2*).

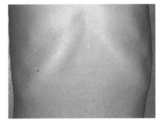

Fig. 1.2: Harrison's sulcus, seen in those with chronic respiratory conditions. Note the flaring of the costal margin with an inferior groove.

Palpation

- Trachea central?
- Assess chest expansion as you would in adults. In children ≈ ≥5 years; 3–5cm is normal.
- Tactile vocal fremitus can be assessed – older children will be able to say '99' as in adults, but in younger children this won't be possible. If they are crying, you can use this instead.

Percussion

- Do sensitively, but essentially the same as in adults – particularly in children of school age.

Auscultation

- If you do not have a paediatric diaphragm on your stethoscope, it is best to use the bell for auscultation of the younger child's chest.
- Auscultate in the traditional way, listening for equality of air entry, vesicular vs. bronchial breath sounds and any added sounds (such as wheeze or crackles / rales).
  - It is common in children to hear 'transmitted upper airway sounds'. These are sounds from the upper respiratory tract that are 'transmitted' into the chest so that you hear them on auscultation – these tend to be loud, inspiratory, coarse and are heard diffusely throughout the chest. They are usually a sign of an upper respiratory tract infection.

1.2.4 Gastrointestinal

Inspection

- Inspect the abdomen for any **s**kin changes, **s**cars, **s**welling or a**s**ymmetry.
- There are some normal variants in children:
  - A protuberant abdomen is normal in toddlers.
  - Umbilical hernias are not unusual, particularly in black infants.
  - Rectus divarication is sometimes seen and is normal (see *Fig. 1.3*).
- Inspect the buttocks for any wasting – indicates recent weight loss.
- **Always** check the hernial orifices.

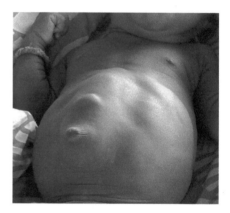

Fig. 1.3: Rectus divarication.

Palpation

- It is imperative that the abdomen is relaxed – you may find the child more compliant if you have them stand up, although lying down is optimal.
- Palpate the nine regions of the abdomen for tenderness or masses.
  - Is the mass indentable? If so, this is usually just faeces, particularly if it is found in the left iliac fossa.
- Liver:
  - As in an adult, moving from the right iliac fossa to the right hypochondrium. It is usually palpable 1–2cm below the right costal margin ≤2 years old.

- Spleen:
  - As with adults, starting in the right iliac fossa and moving to the left hypochondrium. It is sometimes palpable in infants, protruding 1–2cm below the left costal margin. Characteristically, spleens move with respiration, have a notched lateral border and you cannot get above them.
- Kidney:
  - Ballot as normal.
- Bladder:
  - **Is** palpable in neonates and infants. This is normal.

Percussion

- Percuss for the liver and spleen as normal.
- Ascites:
  - Shifting dullness is of far higher utility than fluid thrill. To do this, percuss from the midline to the flank, stopping **as soon** as you hear a dull percussion note. Keeping your finger in the same place, roll the child onto their opposite side and leave them there for ≥30 seconds. Percuss in this spot again – if it was ascitic fluid, the percussion note will now be resonant rather than dull.

Auscultation

- Listen for bowel sounds and bruit.

1.2.5 Cardiovascular

Inspection

- Sweatiness / clamminess – may be a sign of cardiac failure.
- Jugular venous pressure – not usually visible in children.
- Inspect the chest for:
  - Any **s**kin changes, **s**cars, **s**welling or a**s**ymmetry
  - Ventricular impulse – seen in thin children commonly, but may represent ventricular enlargement.

Palpation

- Pulse rate – usually done at the **brachial** artery. This is most easily elicited by having the arm fully extended and palpating medial to the insertion of the biceps brachii.
  - Brachio-femoral / radio-femoral delay – signs of coarctation of the aorta.
- Apex beat, heaves and thrills as in an adult.
- Right ventricular enlargement – a parasternal heave is felt. Place the fingertips along the left sternal edge (approx. 2nd to 4th intercostal spaces) to elicit.

Percussion

- Nil.

Auscultation

- Use the **bell** in younger children.
- Particularly with young children, it can be difficult to ascertain where a murmur is in the cardiac cycle due to their fast heart rates. You may find palpating the brachial pulse useful.
- As with adults.
  - Heart sounds: S2 may be physiologically split in children and a third heart sound (S3) is **not** always pathological.
  - Murmurs: if a murmur is heard, it is best to then listen in all areas with both the diaphragm and the bell. The difficulty lies in distinguishing if this is an 'innocent' (aka 'flow') murmur – heard in ≤50% of children – or pathological. Their distinguishing features are described in the box above.
    - The severity of murmurs is graded with the Levine scale – see *Table 1.4*.

Characteristics of innocent murmurs
Changes with position and respiration
Soft (grade 1–3)
Systolic
Short duration

Table 1.4: The Levine scale

Grade	Description	Thrill
1	Quiet, but definite	–
2	Soft	–
3	Easily heard	–
4	Loud	+
5	Very loud	+
6	Loudest	+

1.2.6 Neurological

Neurological examination of the infant is technically challenging and probably beyond the scope of a FY1's competence. Once into early childhood, when the child is able to follow basic instruction, you will be able to perform the examination as you would on an adult. We therefore only lay out what is required *in addition to* the 'full' neurological examination, as well as some additional examination techniques in the infant.

Inspection – both infants and school-age children

- Dysmorphic features and abnormal facies.
- Movement – do they move **spontaneously**? Are there any abnormal movements? Tremor?
- Walking:
  - How do they stand up? Is the Gower sign (*Fig. 1.4*) present (the patient uses their hands to 'walk' up their legs to push them into the standing position – seen in Duchenne muscular dystrophy (DMD))?

- Stiffness?
- Waddling ('Trendelenburg') gait? – seen in spastic diplegia (a form of cerebral palsy), DMD and developmental dysplasia of the hip.
- Ataxia?
- Muscle wasting?
- Posture?

Tone – for infants (see *Fig. 1.5*)

- **Position** – hypotonic in the 'frog' position, with hips abducted and arms extended? Hypertonic with extended legs that are crossed ('scissoring')?
- Hold their arms and pull them into the sitting position – is there **head lag** beyond 4/12 age (hypotonic)?
- Ventral suspension – now pick the infant up with your hand on the child's abdomen. Do they droop over your hand (hypotonic)? Are they stiff (hypertonic)?
- Next, put one of your hands in each of the child's axillae and pick them up – do they feel like they're floppy and going to slip through your hands (hypotonic)?
- You can also assess tone as you would in an adult.

Power – for infants

- Most of your information will come from observation – are they moving spontaneously? Are they performing anti-gravity movements (i.e. lifting head up or raising arms / legs from the bed)?

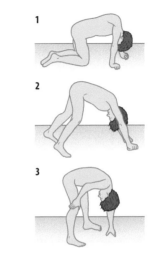

Fig. 1.4: Gower sign.

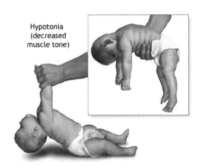

Fig. 1.5: A hypotonic infant with excessive / delayed head lag and floppiness in ventral suspension.

OSCE tips: Gradation of muscular power	
Grade	**Description**
5	Normal power. The muscle is able to move the joint through a full range of movement (ROM) against full resistance from the examiner
4	Muscle able to move joint through full ROM but at reduced resistance
3	Full ROM against gravity but not against any resistance from the examiner
2	Full ROM only with gravity eliminated
1	Muscle contraction seen or palpable, but no movement achieved
0	No movement and muscular contraction seen / felt

Coordination – for school-age chidren

- Assess pronator drift as in adults.
- Upper limb: observe the child playing. Ask them to undo / redo their buttons. Ask them to build a tower of bricks.
- Lower limb: ask them to walk heel–toe. Ask them to hop, skip and run.

Reflexes – infants

- Use a small tendon hammer to elicit the reflexes as in an adult (see *Table 1.5*).
- Babinski reflex (the plantar reflex) may be upgoing to the age of ~8/12; however, it is unreliable and unpleasant so not necessarily needed as part of the examination (see *Fig. 1.6*).
- Test for clonus.

Table 1.5: Nerve roots of the deep tendon reflexes (main nerve root is in bold)

Reflex	Nerve roots
Achilles (calcaneal) tendon	**S1**/S2
Patellar tendon	L3/**L4**
Biceps brachii tendon	C5/C6
Brachioradialis tendon	C5/**C6**
Triceps tendon	**C7**/C8

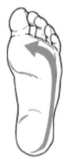

Fig. 1.6: The action required for eliciting the Babinski reflex.

Sensation

- Usually only done crudely – tickle the child and see if they withdraw.
- If a more complete assessment is required, perform as you would in an adult.

Cranial nerves – infants

- In an older, compliant child this examination (see *Fig. 1.7*) can be completed as in adults.
- In neonates and infants, **observation is particularly important**.

I (Olfactory)	• Rarely performed in children.
II (Optic)	• **Visual acuity:** does the child fix on objects? Offer increasingly small objects and see if the child will grasp them. • **Visual fields:** have someone distract the child and shine a light towards their eye from different quadrants → does the child turn their head towards it? • **Pupils:** shine a light → equal and reactive? • Direct ophthalmoscopy (where possible).
III (Oculomotor), IV (Trochlear) and VI (Abducens)	• Look for strabismus. • Does the child spontaneously look in all directions, or are any movements limited? Try to get the child to focus on a toy and follow it. • Doll's head: turn the child's head left and right – their eyes should fix on an object, rather than turning with the head.
V (Trigeminal)	• **Sensation:** does the child respond to touching different areas of the face? • **Motor:** are temporalis and masseter contracting?
VII (Facial)	• Look for facial asymmetry when smiling / crying.
VIII (Vestibulocochlear)	• Strike a tuning fork and place it next to the child's ear → they should turn towards it (in neonates, sudden noises also cause them to briefly freeze).
IX (Glossopharyngeal) and X (Vagus)	• Assess the soft palate and uvula when crying → central or deviated? • Ask the parents about any problems with sucking / feeding.
XI (Accessory)	• Observe the child to see if they turn their head both ways.
XII (Hypoglossal)	• Problems identified with feeding (asked in CN XI and X) may indicate an issue with CN XII also. • Look at the tongue for deviation, wasting and fasciculation.

Fig. 1.7: Cranial nerve examination.

1.2.7 ENT

Ears

- Begin by assessing the ears from the front – are they **low set** (the superior-most part of the helix is lower than a horizontal line drawn from the palpebral fissures) or **protruding** (bilaterally – 'bat ears' due to absence of the anti-helix, or unilaterally – suspect mastoiditis).
- **Correctly position the child:** have them at 90° to their parent, sitting on their leg, with the child's legs sandwiched between the parent's thighs. The parent uses one arm to gently (but firmly) grasp around the child's thorax and arms, whilst the other parental arm is placed on the side of the child's head, which is then pulled against the parental chest.
- Hold the auroscope **like a pen**, using your right hand to look in the right ear and vice versa. Rest your little finger against the child's head so that, should they flinch, you are *preventing the auroscope from entering the auditory canal too deeply*.
- Pull the pinna upwards in infants and downwards in older children.
- **Inspect** the auditory canal as you enter with the auroscope.
- Check the **tympanic membrane**, looking at its **colour** (normal = grey / white with good light reflex), **continuity** (perforations), **contour** (bulging vs. retracted) and anything **behind it**.

Nose

- Begin by **inspecting** the nose externally for any abnormalities or **discharge**.
- **Listen** for noisy breathing sounds, indicative of a partially obstructed nasal passage.
- **Feel** for exit of air from the nares (nostrils) by placing a fingertip under each one. An alternative is to place a mirror or metallic spatula underneath and look for misting.
- **Gently lift the tip** of the nose and inspect the anterior nares for any obvious abnormalities.
- Place the tip of the auroscope (with its *largest attachment*) gently into the nares.
  - Look for any nasal **mucosa changes**, polyps or blood. Occasionally, a foreign body will be found.

Throat

- *Leave this until the very end of all of your examinations*, as a non-compliant child – who does not readily open their mouth wide – will often become distressed by this examination. It is worth mentioning this to the parent and reassuring them that it is not painful for their child.
- **Position:** only needed if the child is refusing to have their throat examined. Have the child sitting facing you on their parent's lap. One parental arm holds their thorax and arms, whilst the other is placed against the child's forehead and the head pulled gently against the parent's chest.
- In general, the opportunity to examine the tonsils and pharynx **will be fleeting** so make sure that you have a good, bright light ready.
- Ask the child to open their mouth as wide as they can. This may be enough for you to visualize what you need to but, if not, use a **wooden spatula** to gently depress the tongue.
- **Pharynx** – erythema or other mucosal changes.
- Tonsils – their **colour**, **exudate** and if they are grossly enlarged (meeting in the midline).
- Tongue – size, colour and any coating.
- **Oral mucosa** – particularly of the palate, where you may see evidence of a cleft, or mucosal changes found in some infections (such as Koplik spots in measles).

Chapter 2

Development and its assessment

2.1 Growth and puberty

Physiology

A child's growth is determined by a number of factors:

- **Genetic potential** – a child of small parents will often be small itself.
- Sufficient **nutritional intake** – may be limited by parental health beliefs or poverty.
- Appropriate **endocrine regulation** of growth.
- **Co-morbidities** – children with chronic health problems are often smaller.
- **Emotional health** – if a child is neglected or understimulated, they may not grow to their genetic potential.

Assessment of growth

In the UK, growth is assessed by measuring **height** (>2 y/o) or **length** (<2 y/o), **weight** and **head circumference** (in infants). This is plotted on the **UK-WHO chart**. There are different charts for girls, boys and trisomy 21, available from the Royal College of Paediatrics and Child Health website at www.rcpch.ac.uk.

> **Prematurity should be corrected for** until the age of **2 years**.
>
> For example, if you see a 4-month-old baby that was born at 32 weeks' gestation, you would plot that at 2 months on the chart (as the baby was born 8 weeks early).

> Children's **centiles should be tracked** from birth.
>
> If ≥2 **centile lines are crossed** concerns should be raised and the child investigated for a cause.

OSCE tips: Important numbers to know for normal growth	
Weight	It's **acceptable for babies to lose 10%** of their birthweight in the first 10 days **of life**
	Babies should have **doubled** their weight by **4 months** and tripled it by 1 year
Length	Birth length is typically **doubled** at **4 years** of age
Head circumference	~35cm at birth and increases roughly 1cm a month for the first year

Normal puberty

Puberty in females (see Fig. 2.1)

- Average age 11 years (range 8–13).
- Order of development: **thelarche** (breast development) → **adrenarche** (pubic hair) → **menarche** (menstruation).
- Takes on average 4–5 years to complete.
- Average age of menarche is 12.5 years.

Puberty in males

- Begins on average **18 months later** than girls.
- Tanner staging is used to assess growth of the testes and penis as well as adrenarche (pubic hair development).
- Puberty is said to have begun once the **testicular volume reaches 4ml**.

Precocious puberty

Hx
- Puberty is deemed precocious if **secondary sexual characteristics** (i.e. features of puberty) develop at **<8 years in girls** and **<9 years in boys**.
- **Central** (GnRH dependent) – due to abnormal activation of the hypothalamic–pituitary–gonadal axis (HPGA): **normal puberty happening too early**.
- **Peripheral** (GnRH independent) – does not involve the HPGA: **abnormal puberty being triggered by something independent of the normal axis**.

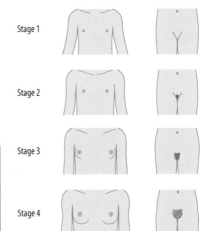

Stage 1

Stage 2

Stage 3

Stage 4

Stage 5

Fig. 2.1: Stages of puberty in females.

DDx
- **Central** – constitutional / familial early puberty; **intracranial tumour**; idiopathic.
- **Peripheral** – endocrine disorders; hormone-secreting **adrenal tumours**; McCune–Albright syndrome.

Ix
- **Imaging – brain MRI** to rule out central tumour.
- **USS ovaries / testes** to assess size and presence of gonadal tumours.
- **Endocrine** – serum gonadotrophin and sex steroid (oestrogen, testosterone) levels.

Management

- **Precocious or delayed puberty should be investigated** because:
  - sinister causes need to be ruled out and
  - the psychological impact for the child may be significant.
- Precocious puberty is managed with **GnRH analogues** that cause a significant drop in gonadotrophin levels.

Developmental assessment

The purpose of this assessment is to determine whether the child's **neurodevelopmental performance** is similar to another child of their age. The 'key' skills are termed **milestones**.

Milestones are accrued:

1. in a **consistent, predictable** sequence
2. at **variable** times; however, this variability may be narrow (e.g. smiling) or wide (e.g. crawling)
3. **within an upper limit**, after which absence of the skill is always abnormal (→ Red Flag).

The assessment is categorized into four broad groups of skills that are evaluated, as shown in *Tables 2.1–2.4*.

Table 2.1: Gross motor skills			
	Time	**Skill (gross motor)**	Red Flag **(upper limit)**
Head control	6w	Develops head control	
	4–6m	No head lag when pulled to sit	No head control (6m)
Movement	6m	Sits ± support	
	9m	Can sit alone ± crawling (varies widely)	Cannot sit unsupported (12m)
	10m	Pulls to stand	
	12m	Cruises ± walking	Not weight-bearing (12m)
	18m	Walks confidently	Not walking (18m)
	2y	Kicks ball and runs	Not running (2.5y)

Table 2.2: Fine motor and visual skills			
	Time	**Skill (fine motor)**	Red Flag **(upper limit)**
Dexterity	3m	Holds object in palm	Does not hold object in hand (5m)
	6m	Transfers object from hand to hand	
Manipulation	9m	Immature pincer grip	
	12m	Mature pincer grip	
Bricks	18m	Stacks 2–4 bricks + hand dominance	
Pencil	2y	Straight line	
	3y	Draws circle	
	4y	Draws cross	
	5y	Draws triangle	

Table 2.3: Speech and language skills

Time	Skill (speech and language)	Red Flag (upper limit)
3m	Turns to sound	No response to stimuli (3m)
3–6m	Vocalizations	
9m	Double syllable babble (e.g. 'baba' or 'mama')	No babble (9m)
12m	2–3 words with meaning	
18m	~10 words with meaning	No words (18m)
2y	Links 2 words together	Cannot join 2 words (2y)
3y	Short, full sentences	Cannot speak in full sentences (3y)

Table 2.4: Social skills

Time	Skills (social)	Red Flag (upper limit)
6w	First smile	
3m	Laughs out loud	
9m	Waves goodbye	No gestures (12m)
12m	Stranger anxiety	
18m	Spoon-feeds self and imitative play (e.g. everyday activities)	No symbolic play (18m)
3y	Dresses self and toilet trained (highly variable)	

Causes of developmental delay

Developmental delay may be **global** (all domains affected) or **specific** (i.e. just a single domain), and the aetiologies are broad.

	Antenatal	Perinatal and postnatal
Global delay	• Genetic: Down syndrome; neurofibromatosis; fragile X; Duchenne muscular dystrophy; tuberous sclerosis; many others • Metabolic and endocrine: hypothyroidism; PKU; MCAD; others • Toxins: drugs and alcohol	• Infection • Trauma / brain injury → cerebral palsy • Neglect

Specific delay	Gross motor	Fine motor and vision	Speech and language	Social skills
	• Spina bifida or cerebral palsy	• Retinoblastoma • Retinopathy of prematurity	• Hearing problems (i.e. otitis media with effusion, deafness of any cause)	• Autistic spectrum disorder • Fragile X

Chapter 3

Neonatal medicine

Normal neonatal physiology and anatomy

An understanding of foetal physiology and the transitions that must occur after birth to allow survival will allow you to better appreciate newborn disease and management.

Pathophysiology

Circulation

In utero, the foetal circulation acts to **bypass** the lungs, as the placenta already provides oxygenated blood. A sequence of changes occur in the peripartum period which then switch the function of oxygenation from the placenta to the lungs.

There are 4 shunts *in utero*, labelled in *Fig. 3.1*:

a) Ductus venosus (bypassing the liver)

b) Foramen ovale (between the left and right atria)

c) Ductus arteriosus (between the pulmonary artery and the aorta)

d) Placenta.

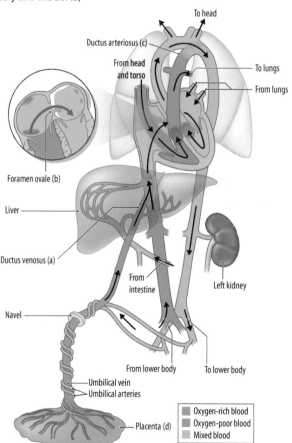

Fig. 3.1: Foetal circulation.

Steps in foetal circulation

1. **Oxygenated blood** is carried through the **umbilical vein**. It enters the foetal circulation via the **ductus venosus (a)** into the **inferior vena cava (IVC)**, distal to where the IVC has given a supply of blood to the liver.
2. The IVC drains into the right atrium. Here, the **foramen ovale (b)** is patent: this shunts most (but not all) blood from right → left atrium (because, *in utero*, **the right-sided pressure is greater than on the left**). Shunted blood therefore **bypasses the lungs.**
3. Some blood remains in the right side of the heart, so leaving via the pulmonary artery. Blood flows through the **patent ductus arteriosus (c)** between pulmonary artery and aorta; again, **bypassing the lungs.**
4. **Deoxygenated blood** flows back to **the placenta (d)** via the **umbilical arteries.**

Circulation changes during birth

1. Removal of placenta
2. Onset of breathing
3. Rapid reduction in pulmonary vascular resistance
4. Closure of shunts (ductus arteriosus, ductus venosus, foramen ovale).

The physiology for these circulatory changes is as follows:

- The amniotic fluid in the lungs is displaced by **squeezing** within the **birth canal**.
- Onset of breathing **increases PaO$_2$** and normalizes pH and PaCO$_2$. These induce pulmonary vasodilatation and therefore **reduce pulmonary resistance**.
- **Clamping the umbilical cord** immediately **increases systemic vascular resistance**.
- The increase in systemic pressure means the **left atrial pressure now exceeds the right atrial pressure** → the foramen ovale closes.
- The **increase in PaO$_2$** triggers closure of the ductus arteriosus within the first day of life.

Gastrointestinal (GI) tract

- Develops as a tube from 6 weeks' gestation.
- The **foetus swallows amniotic fluid** from **16 weeks' gestation** and this is where **proteins (including antibodies providing passive immunity)** from the mother are transferred to the foetus.
- Nutrients can be **absorbed via the gut from 25 weeks' gestation**, although transit time is much slower in low gestation babies.
- **Coordination of suck-and-swallow** (necessary for adequate feeding after birth) develops after **34 weeks' gestation.**

Hepatic function

- *In utero*, the neonatal liver has little function; **toxin filtering and metabolism are performed by the placenta**.
- After birth, the liver starts to adjust to its new function but will not be at full capacity for a **few months**.
  - **Neonatal drugs** often need to be given at lower doses or increased intervals because of the **immaturity in metabolic function.**

Newborn examination

All newborns should have a formal examination **within the first 24 hours of life** prior to discharge. This is done to screen for major abnormalities, to elicit any concerns from the parents and get baseline centile measurements.

Epidemiology and risk factors

- A major congenital abnormality is present in **0.1–0.2% of live births**; it is important to remember that not all will be apparent in the first day of life.
- Incidence doubles in children of consanguineous parents.
- Incidence is also higher with increasing maternal age and lower socio-economic status.

Investigation and diagnosis

Hx
- General appearance and skin colour?
- How is infant handling? Sleepy? Crying? Floppy?
- Have midwives or parents raised any concerns?
- How is parent–infant relationship developing?
- Weight? Length? Head circumference?
- Any complications at birth?
- APGAR scores?
- Maternal mental and physical health history?

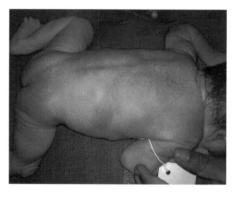

Fig. 3.2: A newborn with multiple Mongolian blue spots including over the sacrum (classical positioning). It is very common in infants of Afro-Caribbean or Asian descent.

Ex
- Examination should be done in a top to toe, systematic fashion; see *Clinical features*, below.
- It is imperative that **Mongolian blue spots** and other **birthmarks** are clearly **documented** at birth as they can often look like bruises and may lead to false accusations of child abuse (see *Fig. 3.2*).

Ix
- Dependent on findings.
- The heel prick (**Guthrie** card) on **day 5 of life** screens for common illnesses (sickle cell anaemia, cystic fibrosis, congenital hypothyroidism and common metabolic defects: PKU/MCADD/MSUD/IVA/GA1/HCU).
- Congenitally **dislocated hips** require **ultrasound.**

DDx
- The **vast majority of newborn infants are well** but it is important to have a high level of clinical suspicion to pick up illness in this age group. A **common problem is sepsis** but keep in mind the possibility of a **congenital defect** or **inborn error of metabolism.**

Clinical features assessed in the newborn examination

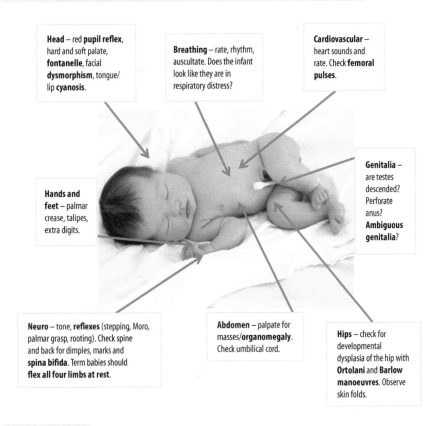

Head – red **pupil reflex**, hard and soft palate, **fontanelle**, facial **dysmorphism**, tongue/lip **cyanosis**.

Breathing – rate, rhythm, auscultate. Does the infant look like they are in respiratory distress?

Cardiovascular – heart sounds and rate. Check **femoral pulses**.

Genitalia – are testes descended? Perforate anus? **Ambiguous genitalia**?

Hands and feet – palmar crease, talipes, extra digits.

Neuro – tone, **reflexes** (stepping, Moro, palmar grasp, rooting). Check spine and back for dimples, marks and **spina bifida**. Term babies should **flex all four limbs at rest**.

Abdomen – palpate for masses/**organomegaly**. Check umbilical cord.

Hips – check for developmental dysplasia of the hip with **Ortolani** and **Barlow manoeuvres**. Observe skin folds.

Management

- Dependent on examination findings.
- Most newborn examinations you do will be normal, so it is important to be vigilant for subtle abnormalities.

OSCE tips 1: The newborn examination

- Document any birthmarks.
- Plot newborn on growth chart.
- Get senior input if you are unsure of any findings.
- Ask Mum how she is feeling and if she has any concerns.

Immunization schedule

The aim of immunization in childhood is to **prevent disease** and to allow for 'herd immunity' within the population. Vaccines may be **live attenuated** viruses, **inactivated** or **killed viruses** or **components of bacteria**. *Table 3.1* shows current UK schedule.

Table 3.1: UK immunization schedule (autumn 2018)

Age due/diseases protected against	Birth	2 months	3 months	4 months	12–13 months	3 years 4 months	12–13 years	14 years	*
BCG	At risk								
HepB	At risk								
Hib									
PCV									
MenB									
Rotavirus									
MenC									
MMR									
DTaP/IPV									
HPV (girls)									
Td/IPV									
MenACWY									
Influenza									

BCG – Bacillus Calmette–Guérain (for TB); D – diphtheria; Hep – hepatitis; Hib – *Haemophilus influenzae* type b; HPV – human papillomavirus; IPV – polio; Men – meningitis; MMR – measles, mumps, rubella; P – pertussis; PCV – pneumococcal vaccine; T – tetanus; * – eligible age groups. Note that several vaccines can be combined into one single vaccination.

Diagnosis and investigation

Hx   **Contraindications – anaphylaxis** to previous vaccine or vaccine component; anaphylaxis to egg (influenza and yellow fever only); **immunocompromise** (live vaccines only); **acute illness** with **fever** and systemic upset.

Ex   Common **side-effects** – low grade **fever; swelling** of injection site. Anaphylaxis is very rare.

There is **no link between the MMR vaccine and autism** and parents should be reassured as such.

Prematurity and intrauterine growth restriction

Birthweight (low or very low, referred to as LBW or VLBW, respectively) and **intrauterine growth restriction** (IUGR) (see *OSCE tips 2*) have a significant impact on neonatal morbidity and mortality.

Epidemiology and risk factors

- **Perinatal mortality rate** = number of stillbirths and neonatal deaths within **first week of life**, per 1000 live births.
- **Neonatal mortality rate** = total deaths per 1000 live births in **first 28 days**.
- Current stillbirth rate is 3.87:1000 (2015); neonatal mortality rate is 1.4:1000.
- **7% of live births** are premature or LBW in the UK.

IUGR can be broadly categorized into two distinct types (see box below) – symmetrical and asymmetrical. The former tends to follow an insult **early in pregnancy**, whereas the latter is due to **late** insults.

Table 3.2: Risk factors for prematurity/IUGR
Multiple pregnancy
Maternal illness
Placental insufficiency
In utero infection
Genetic disorder

Types of IUGR	
Symmetrical IUGR (~25%)	**Asymmetrical IUGR (~75%)**
• Proportionally small head, length and weight • Why? Intrauterine infections and chromosomal abnormalities	• Small length and weight, with a preserved head size; usually due to hypoxia • Why? Maternal or placental issues, such as placental insufficiency or pre-eclampsia

Diagnosis and investigation

Hx Ask about maternal health, pregnancy complications and any previous pregnancies. **Were any concerns raised on antenatal scans?**

Ex Dependent on how premature the infant is. Examine for **dysmorphism** (although difficult in very premature babies). Congenital anomalies are more common in this group.

Ix Dependent on infant's specific issues. **Blood gas** at delivery is typical, to get baseline of how unwell infant is.

OSCE tips 2: Definitions

- **Prematurity** – any birth before 37/40 gestation
- **IUGR** – failure of the foetus to achieve genetic growth potential
- **SGA** (small for gestational age) – a newborn below a certain centile for that particular gestation, usually but not always the 10th centile
- **LBW** – a newborn weighing less than 2500g
- **VLBW** – a newborn weighing less than 1500g
- **Stillbirth** – a foetus born after 24/40 that never shows any signs of life
- **Neonatal death** – death of a newborn within 28 days of delivery

Management

- Should be managed in **NICU** (neonatal intensive care). Very premature infants often require **intubation**, **ventilation** and **surfactant**.
- Often need feeding support and to be closely monitored for complications (see *Section 3.5*).

Pathophysiology

Neonates have thin skin, little adipose tissue and a large body surface area comparative to their body weight; they are therefore **very susceptible to heat loss** and consequent **hypothermia**.

Epidemiology and risk factors

- Hypothermia can develop quickly in preterm and unwell neonates.
- Hypothermia leads to a significant **increase in morbidity and mortality** in the newborn period and should be aggressively avoided.
- For risk factors see *Table 3.3*.

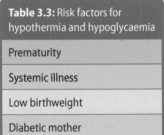

Table 3.3: Risk factors for hypothermia and hypoglycaemia
Prematurity
Systemic illness
Low birthweight
Diabetic mother

 Hypothermia may indicate neonatal sepsis and always requires assessment of the baby.

Management

Babies lose heat **through convection, conduction, evaporation and radiation** (*Fig. 3.3*). This should be combatted by:
- Warm mattress / skin to skin with Mum (conduction)
- Keeping room temperature warm and avoiding draughts (convection)
- Wrapping baby, including hat and socks (evaporation)
- Using incubator as radiant heat source (radiation)

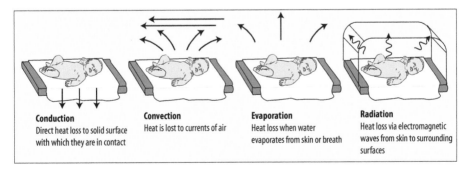

Conduction
Direct heat loss to solid surface with which they are in contact

Convection
Heat is lost to currents of air

Evaporation
Heat loss when water evaporates from skin or breath

Radiation
Heat loss via electromagnetic waves from skin to surrounding surfaces

Fig. 3.3: Physiology or types of neonatal heat loss.

3.5.2 Hypoglycaemia

Pathophysiology

Hypoglycaemia (blood sugar <2.6mmol/L) is a common problem in newborns and has four broad causes: ↓ glucose **production** (e.g. preterms, metabolic errors), ↑ **glucose demands** (sepsis, hypothermia), **hyperinsulinism** (diabetic mother) or **endocrine** problems.

Epidemiology and risk factors

- Hypoglycaemia is common and often transient.
- For risk factors see *Table 3.3.*

Diagnosis and investigation

Hx	**Size** (small or macrosomic), jaundiced? Polycythaemic? Observe for **apnoeas**. May show **neurological signs of hypoglycaemia** (floppy, jittery, irritable, **seizures**). Any **dysmorphic** features? **Ambiguous genitalia** suggesting endocrine cause?

Ex	May be asymptomatic ∴ **low threshold to check infants** of diabetic mothers or those feeding poorly. Symptoms include **jitteriness**, hypotonia, **apnoeas ± seizures** (severe).

Ix	Check blood sugars and temperature regularly in NICU/SCBU settings. If identified investigate driving cause. **Symptomatic** or severe (**<1.5mmol/L**) hypoglycaemia in a newborn should prompt a **'hypo screen'**. This looks for endocrine and metabolic causes.

Management

- **1.6–2.6mmol/L and asymptomatic** – feed infant and consider increasing feed frequency and volume. Most hypoglycaemic episodes are transient with no sinister cause.
- **Severe (<1.6mmol/L) or symptomatic** – treat immediately with IV dextrose (10%), admit to neonatal unit and monitor blood sugars hourly until stable. These children require a 'hypo screen', which aims to identify the **common endocrine and metabolic aetiologies** of paediatric hypoglycaemia.

3.5.3 Respiratory distress syndrome

Respiratory distress syndrome (RDS), also known as **hyaline membrane disease**, is a condition of prematurity caused by **insufficient levels of surfactant**; consequently, it is more prevalent the more premature an infant is. It manifests in a **tachypnoeic** newborn showing signs of respiratory distress.

Pathophysiology

Lack of surfactant in the lungs may be because the infant is **premature** (→ produced in the final trimester) or because its effect has been **inhibited by asphyxia**. Surfactant **lowers alveolar surface tension** allowing the lungs to open and close easily without fully collapsing. Loss of surfactant results in **alveolar collapse**, and the cycle shown in *Fig. 3.4* ensues.

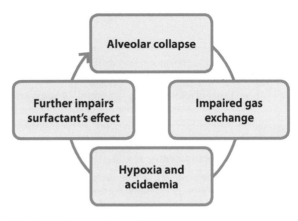

Fig. 3.4: Pathophysiology of RDS.

Epidemiology and risk factors

Table 3.4: Risk factors for RDS	
Prematurity	• The most important risk factor. The more premature the infant, the higher the risk of RDS.
Perinatal asphyxia	• Difficult birth. • Meconium aspiration. • Sepsis. • Congenital lung anomalies.
Maternal diabetes	• Lungs are delayed in their maturity.

Clinical features

Symptoms
- Distressed and unwell infant.
- Poor feeding.

Signs
- **Tachypnoea** (>60 breaths per minute).
- Hypoxia.
- **Respiratory distress** (intercostal and subcostal recession, head bobbing, tracheal tug, nasal flaring).
- **Grunting** (in an attempt to increase airway pressure and open collapsed alveoli).

OSCE tips 3: Surfactant treatment in premature babies

- Surfactant is produced by **type II pneumocytes**, which are **present from 20/40 gestation**, but ↑↑ in number during the final trimester.
- All neonates born **<28/40** should get surfactant after delivery, and **maternal antenatal steroids** should be given.
- Treatment with exogenous surfactant in RDS **reduces mortality by 40%**.

Investigation and diagnosis

Hx
- Usually a premature neonate (although may be full-term baby with a diabetic mother / asphyxia in birth history or a twin / triplet).
- Onset of respiratory distress occurs **<4 hours after birth**.

Ex
- Tachypnoeic (RR >60) ± cyanosis, grunting, intercostal recession and nasal flaring.
- **Reduced air entry** on auscultation.
- May be peripherally oedematous.

Ix
- **Blood gases** (hypoxia + metabolic acidosis).
- **Chest X-ray** (classic changes are of a **ground glass infiltrate** with air bronchograms and reduced lung volume; see *Fig. 3.5*).
- Important to screen for other causes of respiratory distress so send blood cultures, FBC, U&Es and swabs from mother and infant.

DDx
- Sepsis
- Complex heart disease
- Lung hypoplasia
- Pneumothorax
- Severe anaemia

The aim of treatment is to create a homeostatic environment for the neonate to **produce their own surfactant** and thus self-ventilate. This can only happen in the presence of normal pH, temperature and sufficient oxygenation.

Management

1. **Oxygen** to improve oxygenation; aiming for pO_2 between 6 and 10.
2. **Continuous positive airway pressure (CPAP)** and mechanical **ventilation** to give sufficient pressure to open the airways and prevent further lung collapse.
3. **Artificial surfactant** to increase lung compliance and decrease alveolar surface tension.
4. If possible, give **antenatal steroids** to the mother prior to delivery in at-risk pregnancies.
5. Correct hypothermia, acidaemia and hypoglycaemia.

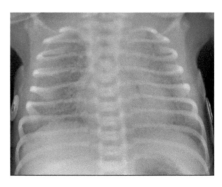

Fig. 3.5: Chest X-ray in RDS. Note the bilateral lung opacification, air bronchograms, small lung volumes and endotracheal tube.

3.5.4 Brain injury

Neurological damage related to prematurity includes **intraventricular haemorrhage** (IVH) and **periventricular leukomalacia** (PVL). Preterm neonates can also develop hypoxic ischaemic encephalopathy (HIE) but this is more commonly associated with neonates born at term and is therefore not covered in this chapter.

Pathophysiology

IVH – alteration in cerebral blood flow (from apnoea / acidaemia / hypotension) results in **bleeding** in the fragile **germinal matrix** (see *Fig. 3.6*); which, if severe enough, will **extend into the ventricles**. The germinal matrix disappears in the third trimester and as such this is a condition seen in neonates born **prior to 32 weeks' gestation** in the vast majority of cases.

PVL – not as well understood as IVH. It is thought that **hypoperfusion** and **excitotoxic cytokines** cause damage to the oligodendroglia, resulting in **white matter injury**.

Epidemiology and risk factors

Table 3.5: Risk factors for brain injury	
VLBW, gestation <32 weeks	• One of the most significant risk factors
Difficult birth, RDS	• Hypoxic episodes during delivery or secondary to lung disease promote release of neurotoxic cytokines
Cardiovascular instability	• Fluctuations in blood pressure affecting cerebral blood flow
Other prematurity complications	• Sepsis and necrotizing enterocolitis cause acidaemia, making the brain more susceptible to injury

Clinical features

Symptoms
- Often asymptomatic, especially if insult is small.
- Seizures and apnoeas may occur with big bleeds.
- Significant neurological insult may present as floppy infant with poor feeding.

Signs
- Abnormal movements or tone may be the only sign of neurological impairment.
- A large IVH may present as a hypovolaemic neonate (tachycardic, peripherally shut down).

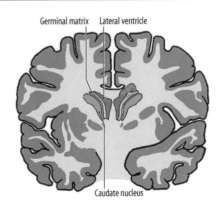

Fig. 3.6: The germinal matrix, the site of injury in IVH. The right side of the diagram shows a bleed into the right lateral ventricle.

33

Investigation and diagnosis

Hx | **IVH** usually occur **within 72 hours** of delivery.

Ask about potential **risk factors** for IVH or PVL; the more risk factors an infant has, the higher the risk of developing a brain injury.

Ex | Examination findings are often subtle or non-existent unless a significant neurological insult has occurred.

DDx | **Subdural** or **subarachnoid** haemorrhage. Hypoxic ischaemic encephalopathy. Seizures secondary to another cause (electrolytes, hypoglycaemia, metabolic).

Ix | Primary investigation for both IVH and PVL is **ultrasound**. This is used to **grade haemorrhages** (IVH) and assess **cystic white matter changes** (PVL). The ultrasound image in *Fig. 3.7* shows cystic changes around the lateral ventricle, as seen in severe PVL.

More subtle white matter changes in PVL are seen on **MRI**.

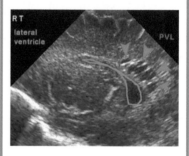

Fig. 3.7: Ultrasound indicating severe PVL.

Management

IVH

- **ABCDE approach**. Optimize airway, ventilate if necessary, keep PO_2 in strict limits, maintain circulatory volume, treat seizures if occur, correct coagulation errors.
- Maintaining good **blood pressure** and **oxygen / carbon dioxide** level control in this vulnerable population reduces the incidence of IVH.

PVL

- Unfortunately once white matter change has occurred there is no treatment to reverse it.
- **Aim is prevention** by, as in IVH, avoiding large blood pressure fluctuations and hypoxia.

OSCE tips 4: Grading IVH

Grade I – isolated to germinal matrix

Grade II – haemorrhage into ventricles, no dilatation of ventricles

Grade III – haemorrhage into ventricle with acute dilatation

Grade IV – parenchymal haemorrhagic infarct

OSCE tips 5: PVL prognosis

Bilateral occipital cystic PVL reliably indicates future development of **spastic diplegia cerebral palsy**.

3.5.5 Infection

Neonatal infections are a significant cause of morbidity and mortality. Sepsis that develops within **72 hours of delivery** is usually of **maternal origin**. After **72 hours** most infections are acquired **from the infant's surroundings** and, in a **premature neonate**, these are often **nosocomial**.

Pathophysiology

- Lack maternal IgG reserves
- Multiple lines *in situ*
- Hospitalized for long periods
- Thin, delicate skin
- Higher incidence of other co-morbidities which predispose to Infection

Epidemiology and risk factors

Note: these risk factors are commonly asked about in exams.

Table 3.6: Risk factors for infection	
• Prematurity • Maternal pyrexia in labour • Premature rupture of membranes (PROM)	• LBW • Long lines *in situ* • Chorioamnioitis • Maternal group B strep colonization

Diagnosis and investigation

Hx
- A clinically **deteriorating** neonate (though signs may be subtle) or **neonatal collapse**.
- Enquire about poor **feeding** (often first sign of illness in babies).
- Presence of one or more **risk factors** significantly increases chance of neonatal infection.
- **Absence of risk factors does not exclude diagnosis of infection.**

Ex
- High index of suspicion important.
- Observations may be deranged; remember, **heart rate and blood pressure changes are LATE signs of sepsis**. Fever is not always present.
- **Auscultate** for **crepitations** / air entry through chest and **bowel sounds**. Palpate for **organomegaly**. Is there a **rash**? Is the **abdomen distended**? Is the **fontanelle sunken** (hypovolaemia) or **bulging** (meningitis)?
- How is the infant handling? Are they **irritable**? Having **seizures**?

Ix	**Septic screen** (nasal / throat / line swabs, bloods, cultures, urine dip, chest X-ray, lumbar puncture, and lines).

DDx	• Congenital infections • Respiratory distress syndrome • Congenital heart defect • Necrotizing enterocolitis

Management

- **Antibiotic** treatment should be commenced **<1 hour if clinical suspicion of infection –** do not delay whilst waiting for investigation results.
- Specific antibiotic regimens will differ but, broadly:
  - **early onset** (<72 hours after birth) – **IV penicillin + IV aminoglycoside**
  - **late onset** (>72 hours after birth) – **IV flucloxacillin + IV aminoglycoside**
  - **plus** acyclovir, to cover for potential herpes simplex virus (HSV) infection.
- Proven infections are treated for at least **7 days**, based on clinical response; **14 days** are required for *Staphylococcus aureus* infections and **21 days for meningitis**. Triple therapy of gentamicin, a broad-spectrum penicillin containing agent and **acyclovir** (to cover for **possible herpes simplex encephalitis**) is typical.

3.5.6 Necrotizing enterocolitis

Necrotizing enterocolitis (NEC) is almost exclusively seen in neonates that have been **orally fed**, although the precise reasons for this are unknown. NEC carries a significant morbidity and mortality burden in premature and low birthweight neonates.

Pathophysiology

Specifics are unknown but **infection** and **ischaemia** occur in the bowel wall with subsequent **inflammatory oedema** and **haemorrhage**. Untreated, this may progress to bowel necrosis and subsequent perforation.

Epidemiology and risk factors

Table 3.7: Risk factors for NEC, seen in up to 20% of VLBW neonates	
Oral feeding (formula higher risk than breast milk)	LBW
Prematurity	VLBW
Other concurrent infection	IUGR
	Perinatal asphyxia

Diagnosis and investigation

Hx
- Classic history is of abdominal **distension** and **bilious aspirates** in a clinically **deteriorating neonate**, with **bloody stools**.
- Usually around **1–2 weeks of age**.

DDx
- Other causes of mechanical intestinal obstruction (i.e. volvulus)
- Congenital bowel malformation
- Hirschsprung disease

Ex
- **Abdominal distension**
- **Vomiting** / bilious aspirates
- Apnoeas, bradycardias
- **Fluctuant temperature**
- Severe untreated NEC may cause neonatal collapse and death.

Ix
- **Abdominal X-ray** (see *Fig. 3.8*)
- Bloods (coagulation, FBC, CRP), blood gases (acidosis).
- Screen for other sources of sepsis.

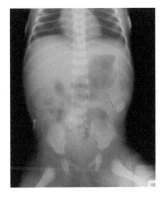

Fig. 3.8: Abdomen X-ray showing **pneumatosis intestinalis** (gas in the bowel wall).

Management

1. Keep infant **nil by mouth**, feed parenterally (**TPN**) and place **nasogastric (NG) tube** for aspirates.
2. **IV antibiotics** (broad-spectrum, to cover aerobic and anaerobic pathogens).
3. Replacement of fluid and electrolyte losses, correction of coagulopathy, oxygenate well.
4. If **bowel perforates** or is not responsive to conservative management, then **laparotomy** ± **bowel resection** is indicated.

3.5.7 Retinopathy of prematurity

Retinopathy of prematurity (ROP) causes significant morbidity even with strict screening in the UK. It is very rare in infants born >32 weeks' gestation or >1500g in weight.

Pathophysiology

- Adequate oxygenation is imperative in the management of premature infants; however, hyperoxygenation is detrimental.

- **Hyperoxygenation inhibits** vascular endothelial growth factor in the retina; subsequent **relative hypoxia** then promotes inappropriate and excessive **blood vessel formation** (see *Fig. 3.9*).
- Untreated, these vessels cause **retinal haemorrhages and scarring** and eventually retinal **detachments**, resulting in visual loss.

Epidemiology and risk factors

- 30% of infants born <1500g develop ROP; we treat 5% and ~1% are left with a significant visual impairment.
- 30% of those treated have a degree of visual impairment.

Table 3.8: Risk factors for ROP
Prematurity
Hyperoxygenation
Low birthweight

Diagnosis and investigation

Hx
- All infants born <32 weeks' gestation or <1500g will be screened in the UK.

Ex
- There is an accepted classification system of stage 1–5 based on the changes seen in the retina on examination (see *OSCE tips 6*).
- Neuro imaging may be indicated if cortical blindness is suspected.

DDx
- Myopia
- Congenital cataract
- Congenital glaucoma
- Cortical blindness

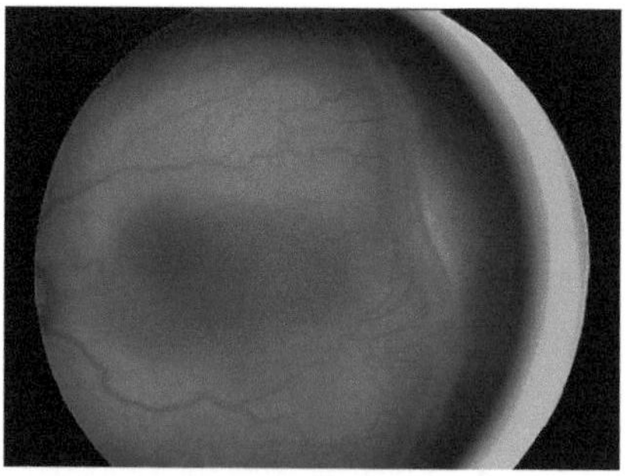

Fig. 3.9: Retinal examination findings. Note dilated vessels and abnormal new vessels developing at the edge of retina.

OSCE tips 6: ROP stages

1. Mild abnormal vessel growth
2. Moderately abnormal vessel growth
3. Severely abnormal vessel growth
4. Partial retinal detachment
5. Complete retinal detachment

Management

- Keep oxygen saturations 90–95% and aim to avoid big swings in oxygenation.
- **Stage 1 and 2 will resolve independently**.
- Those with **stage 3 or above** ROP need **laser treatment** of the peripheral retina to prevent further vessel growth.

Neonatal conditions

Neonatal jaundice

Jaundice is a seen in **≤80% of term and preterm infants**. It's important to appreciate, as high levels of **unconjugated bilirubin cross the blood–brain barrier** (BBB) and cause permanent damage to neural tissue, termed **kernicterus** (bilirubin-induced brain damage). **Onset within 24 hours should be treated as an emergency**.

The most important question is whether the jaundice is **conjugated or unconjugated** as this helps narrow the DDx (see *Table 3.9*).

Pathophysiology

- To understand jaundice you first need to understand bilirubin metabolism and why this makes newborns more susceptible to jaundice.
- **Bilirubin is a degradation product of haemoglobin**; initially it is broken down into **unconjugated** (or indirect, lipid-soluble) bilirubin. This is **bound to albumin** in the blood and **transported to the liver** where it is **conjugated** via glucuronyl transferase into conjugated (or direct, water-soluble) bilirubin.
- **Conjugated bilirubin** is excreted via the **common bile duct** into the **small intestine**; here some is converted to and excreted as **stercobilinogen** (that colours stools dark). Some is **deconjugated** by gut flora and **reabsorbed enterohepatically** and transported to the **kidneys** where it is excreted as **urobilinogen** or **reconjugated** again via the liver (see *Fig. 3.10*).
- An **excess of unconjugated bilirubin** will **saturate** the available **albumin** and this free lipid-soluble bilirubin can cross the BBB. In sufficient quantities this results in kernicterus; this is described in more detail in the subsection below.

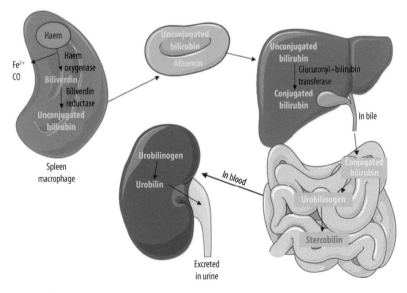

Fig. 3.10: Bilirubin transport.

Newborns are susceptible to high levels of bilirubin because:

1. Their **haemoglobin levels** at birth are high, and foetal haemoglobin lifespan is shorter, leaving a **large source of haemoglobin products to be degraded**.
2. **Hepatic enzymes** are immature or fewer in number and not as efficient at conjugating bilirubin; this is especially true of preterm neonates.
3. **Slow intestinal transit** time causes **deconjugation of bilirubin** and **reabsorption** via the enterohepatic circulation.
4. Many **medications displace bilirubin** from albumin, which contributes to jaundice, especially in **premature infants**.

Table 3.9: Causes of neonatal jaundice	
Conjugated (water-soluble)	**Unconjugated (lipid-soluble)**
Biliary atresia (see later subsection)	Haemolysis (see *OSCE tips 7*)
Hepatitis (viral, neonatal, congenital infection)	Breast milk jaundice (see *OSCE tips 8*)
Cystic fibrosis	Hypothyroidism
Alpha 1 antitrypsin deficiency	Septicaemia
Lipid storage disease	Metabolic disorders – galactosaemia / amino acid disorders / fructosaemia
TPN	Hepatic enzyme defects – Crigler–Najjar, Gilbert syndrome
	Drugs

Epidemiology and risk factors

Table 3.10: Risk factors for neonatal jaundice	
Prematurity	• Immaturity of enzymes allow accumulation of bilirubin. Often polycythaemic which increases bilirubin load.
Breast milk	• Exact physiology unknown, but jaundice seen much more commonly than in formula-fed infants.
Family history	• Again, physiology unknown but a well recognized link.

Clinical features

Symptoms

- Look for symptoms suggestive of an infective cause.
- Neurological symptoms indicate kernicterus.

Signs

- **Yellow skin and sclera** (it is not possible to accurately assess level of bilirubin from how jaundiced a child looks; you must get laboratory levels).
- Hepatomegaly (hepatic, infective or metabolic causes).
- **Hepatosplenomegaly** (haemolytic causes).
- **Pallor**/pale conjunctiva (if haemolytic cause).

OSCE tips 7: Haemolytic jaundice

- Haemolytic disease of the newborn (ABO or rhesus incompatibility)
- G6PD deficiency
- Hereditary spherocytosis
- Alpha thalassaemia

Haemolysis causes an unconjugated hyperbilirubinaemia usually **within first 24 hours of life**. The most severe form is due to **rhesus incompatibility**; however, with routine testing of mothers to see if they are rhesus negative (and giving anti-D prophylaxis if they are), this is now less common. Haemolysis can cause a **very rapid rise** in bilirubin, requiring early treatment.

The **Coombs test** (*Fig. 3.11*) is positive in antibody-mediated haemolytic anaemia (such as ABO or rhesus incompatibility). Antibodies will bind to erythrocyte surface antigens; then when Coombs reagent is added, the presence of the antibodies make the erythrocytes stick together, giving a positive test.

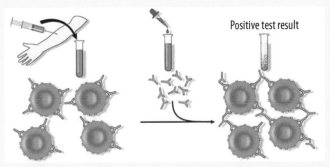

Positive test result

| Blood sample from a patient with immune-mediated haemolytic anaemia: antibodies are shown attached to antigens on the RBC surface | The patient's washed RBCs are incubated with antihuman antibodies (Coombs reagent) | RBCs agglutinate: antihuman antibodies form links between RBCs by binding to the human antibodies on the RBCs |

Fig. 3.11: Direct Coombs test/direct antiglobulin test.

Diagnosis and investigation

Hx
- Ask about **birth history** and **feeding** (Breast or formula? Feeding well?)
- **Time of onset** is very important, as is whether the child was previously well.
- Ask about **stool and urine colour**.
  - **Pale stools and dark urine suggest an obstructive cause**.
- Is there a **family history** of neonatal jaundice or haemolytic disease? What is the **mother's blood group**? Did she have anti-D during pregnancy?
- Is there a possibility of **congenital infection**?
- Is there a history pointing to other infection? (respiratory distress, urinary tract infection (UTI)).

Ex
- **Observations** – are they pyrexial? Tachycardic? Tachypnoeic? **Well or unwell?**
- Do they look **clinically jaundiced**? More difficult to assess in darker skin tones. Evident when serum bilirubin >85micromol/L.
- Are they **dehydrated**? This may exacerbate hyperbilirubinaemia.
- Look for **bruising** (will increase haemoglobin product load) and **pallor** (haemolysis).
- Palpate for **hepatosplenomegaly**.
- A thorough **neurological examination** is essential.

Ix
- Investigate babies requiring treatment: those who become jaundiced within 24 hours of life or those <34 weeks' gestation.
- **Bloods** (FBC, LFTs, split bilirubin and levels, U&Es, Coombs test, maternal and newborn blood type, TFTs, blood film for red cell morphology).
- **G6PD screen** (in high risk groups i.e. Mediterranean, Asian or African origin).
- **Urine** should be dipped and tested for **reducing substances**.
- If infection suspected then swabs, urine, blood and cerebrospinal fluid (CSF) **cultures** should be taken.
- **In many cases no cause is identified.**

DDx
- Biliary atresia
- Sepsis
- Normal skin tone

OSCE tips 8: Breast milk jaundice

- The **most common cause** of neonatal jaundice. Glucuronidases present in the gut and in breast milk deconjugate bilirubin, allowing more to be reabsorbed enterohepatically in breastfed babies so their serum unconjugated bilirubin increases and jaundice develops.
- This persists past 14 days (persistent jaundice) in 10–20% in infants.
- **Breast milk jaundice is not an indication to stop breastfeeding.**
- Breast milk jaundice used to be known as physiological jaundice; this term is no longer used because breast milk jaundice can still result in kernicterus.
- Those meeting treatment guidelines respond well to **phototherapy**. Poor response to phototherapy suggests an alternative cause.

Management

- **Conservative** – most jaundiced babies (especially term) do not require treatment. They can have bilirubin monitored to ensure this does not rise above treatment threshold. They may need support with breastfeeding. Dehydration should be addressed.

- **Phototherapy** – phototherapy reduces unconjugated bilirubin. NICE has charts corrected for gestational age to determine at what level treatment is needed (see *Fig. 3.12*).

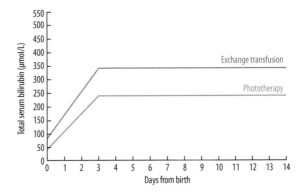

Fig. 3.12: NICE treatment graph for a 34 week gestation baby. The blue line indicates the need for phototherapy and red line for exchange transfusion.

- **Exchange transfusion** – baby's blood volume removed and transfused with donor blood. Indicated with high, **potentially toxic bilirubin levels** or **any signs of kernicterus**. Removes bilirubin, antibodies and corrects anaemia if present. Risk of complications (electrolyte imbalance, volume issues, transfusion reactions).

- **If sepsis suspected as cause, treat urgently.**

3.6.2 Biliary atresia

Pathophysiology

Congenital absence of part or all of the bile duct system. High clinical suspicion and early diagnosis are essential for a good clinical outcome. Without prompt treatment, early hepatic cirrhosis and liver failure will develop. Over 80% are type III (total absence of the bile ducts). *Figure 3.13* shows the different types of biliary atresia.

Epidemiology and risk factors

1 in 14 000 UK live births.

Diagnosis and investigation

Hx
- Often presents with bleeding / bruising associated with jaundice developing within the first 1–2 weeks of life.
- There will be a history of pale stools and dark urine.
- Biliary atresia should be considered in all babies with prolonged jaundice (>14 days).

Ex
- Clinically jaundiced
- Bruising or persistent cephalohaematomas (clotting derangement)

Ix
- **Bloods** (LFTs, GGT, coagulation, viral and metabolic screen), which show a conjugated hyperbilirubinaemia.
- **USS** to look for biliary atresia.
- **Liver biopsy** may be indicated.

DDx Other causes of hyperbilirubinaemia

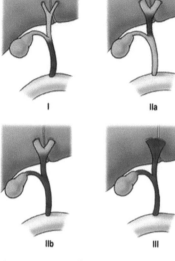

Fig. 3.13: Types of biliary atresia. Note the total absence of bile ducts in type III.

Management

- Biliary atresia is managed with a **Kasai porto-enterostomy** or **liver transplant** (see *Fig. 3.14*).
- Babies with conjugated hyperbilirubinaemia (such as biliary atresia) need extra vitamin K to avoid haemorrhagic disease of the newborn, because their coagulation ability will be impaired.
- Once diagnosis confirmed, urgent discussion is needed with a **tertiary paediatric liver service**.

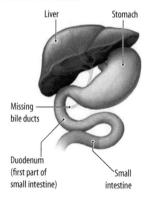

Liver — Stomach

Missing bile ducts

Duodenum (first part of small intestine)

Small intestine

The dotted lines show areas that can be affected by biliary atresia

Stomach

Duodenum (first part of small intestine)

Small intestine connected to liver

During the Kasai procedure, the intestine is attached to the liver. This allows bile to drain

Fig. 3.14: The Kasai procedure.

3.6.3 Kernicterus

Kernicterus is the term used for **bilirubin encephalopathy**.

Pathophysiology

Kernicterus occurs as a result of excess unbound, lipid-soluble, unconjugated bilirubin crossing the BBB. Any illness causing systemic acidosis (such as infection) disrupts the BBB, making kernicterus more likely. The most susceptible areas of the brain are the metabolically active parts with high blood flow – the basal ganglia and the midbrain. If untreated, kernicterus is fatal.

Epidemiology and risk factors

Fortunately now very rare in developed countries.

Table 3.11: Risk factors for kernicterus
High unconjugated bilirubin
Sepsis (makes BBB leaky)
Acidosis (makes brain more susceptible to damage)

Diagnosis and investigation

Hx
- Variable depending on cause of hyperbilirubinaemia.
- Ask about change in newborn's behaviour, tone and feeding.

Ex
- **Acute encephalopathy** – hypotonia, lethargy and poor feeding followed by hypertonia (opisthotonus – see *Fig. 3.15*), irritability and seizures progressing to coma and eventually death if untreated.
- **Longer-term consequences** – cerebral palsy, deafness, intellectual disability.

Ix
- Regular bilirubin levels; it is important to ascertain **how quickly the bilirubin is rising**.
- Aim is prevention and if levels potentially toxic, aggressive and swift intervention.
- Monitor coagulation.

DDx
Other neurological insult (intracranial bleed, infection, ischaemic brain injury)

Management

- Unfortunately **there is no treatment to reverse kernicterus once it has occurred**.
- Management is in **prevention**, aggressive management of potentially toxic bilirubin levels (with **exchange transfusion if any evidence of encephalopathy**).
- Coagulopathy and electrolyte imbalances need correcting.

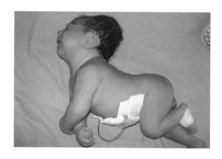

Fig. 3.15: A newborn showing opisthotonus (involuntary arching of the head, neck and spine) due to untreated hyperbilirubinaemia.

3.6.4 Patent ductus arteriosus

Patent ductus arteriosus (PDA) is the abnormal persistence of the duct between the aorta and main pulmonary artery after birth. Ordinarily, the duct should close in the first day of life.

Pathophysiology

- The PDA acts as a left-to-right shunt, as pressure is higher in the aorta than the pulmonary artery. The degree of shunting is dependent on the resistance in the duct.
- With a large shunt congestive heart failure (CHF) develops and, if uncorrected, eventually pulmonary hypertension and eventual reversal of the shunt → cyanosis.
- In premature infants the duct often closes spontaneously, but this is very rare in full-term babies with PDA.

Epidemiology and risk factors

- 5–10% of cases of congenital heart disease (CHD) in term babies.
- 50% of babies born weighing <1500g have significant PDA.

Diagnosis and investigation

Hx
- A small duct will be asymptomatic.
- Larger shunts will have a history of **recurrent chest infections**, failure to thrive and **poor feeding**.
- Older children may present with **exertional dyspnoea**.

Table 3.12: Risk factors for PDA
Prematurity
Cyanotic heart lesion
Female sex
Family history
Chromosomal abnormalities
Maternal drug / alcohol use in pregnancy

Ex
- Classic findings are of a grade 1–4 **continuous 'machinery' murmur**, loudest just below the left clavicle.
- The heart sounds are normal unless pulmonary hypertension is present, when S2 will be loud.
- Examine for **signs of CHF** (tachycardia, tachypnoea, hepatomegaly, poor weight gain).

Ix
- **Chest X-ray (CXR)** – may be normal with a small PDA, but a larger shunt will show cardiac enlargement and increased pulmonary vascular markings.
- **ECG** – large shunts result in ventricular hypertrophy.
- **Echocardiogram** – to investigate size of PDA and if any other structural cardiac defects present (see *Fig. 3.16*).

DDx
- RDS
- Complex cardiac defect
- Sepsis

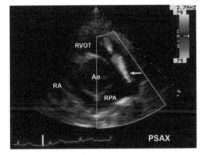

Management

- Closure is indicated if the infant is symptomatic or the PDA is haemodynamically significant.
- Most PDAs are closed via catheter techniques very successfully.
- Surgical ligation is reserved for very large PDAs or those that fail to close following catheter techniques.
- In premature infants, indomethacin or ibuprofen may be used to medically close the duct.
- Medical management of CHF (diuretics).

Fig. 3.16: Echocardiogram. The orange is Doppler of blood flow between pulmonary artery and aorta through a PDA.

3.6.5 Cleft palate and lip

Pathophysiology

A **cleft lip and or palate** (see *Fig. 3.17*) occurs when normal development of facial structures is interrupted *in utero*. The **lip** and nose develop between the **3rd and 7th week** of gestation and the **palate** between the **5th and 12th week**. Interruptions before the 7th week will result in a cleft lip which may extend into the primary (very anterior portion) of the palate. An interruption after the 8th week will result in a cleft of the larger, secondary portion of the palate. **These conditions can occur in isolation or together.**

Epidemiology and risk factors

Table 3.13: Risk factors for cleft lip / palate	
Aneuploidy / genetic syndrome	• Trisomy 18: there are over 300 syndromes associated with a cleft lip / palate.
Family history	• Ethnically, children of Asian descent are at highest risk and Afro-Caribbean heritage the lowest.
Maternal drug use, smoking and alcohol	• Toxin exposure in the first trimester can affect embryological development. Anti-epileptics are a known risk.

Incidence 1:1000 live births. Inheritance is polygenic and not fully understood.

Clinical features

Signs

- Cleft lip (unilateral or bilateral) on examination.
- Cleft palate (check hard palate intact when examining babies) – they may have intact lip but cleft palate.

Symptoms

- **Difficulty establishing feeds.**
- Recurrent **chest infections** (from aspirations).
- **Faltering growth** (from feeding issues).
- If associated with a syndrome, likely to be other multisystem signs and symptoms.

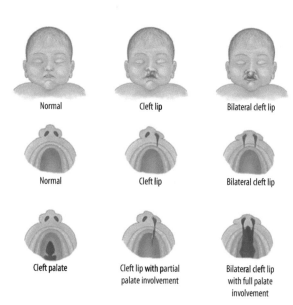

Fig. 3.17: Different grades of cleft lip and palate.

Investigation and diagnosis

Hx
- Ask about **antenatal scans** and **family history**.
- Enquire about **feeding**.
- Smaller cleft palates may only present as **poor feeding**, **faltering growth** or recurrent **chest infections**.

Ex
- Establish whether the problem is **unilateral or bilateral**; gently examine the palate and try to establish how much is involved.
- How effective is the baby's suck? Observe them sucking a finger or pacifier.
- Do a thorough examination looking for other **dysmorphic features**.
- Plot the child on **growth chart**.

Ix
- Larger clefts, especially of the lip, are often picked up on antenatal scans.
- **Genetic testing** to identify presence of a cleft-associated syndrome (of which there are over 300).

DDx
- Pierre Robin sequence
- Part of complex genetic syndrome

Management

Table 3.14: Management of cleft lip / palate

Medical	• Manage as part of an **MDT** at a **tertiary centre** (paediatrician, SALT, maxillofacial surgeon, orthodontist, ENT, cleft specialist nurse, geneticists). • Early involvement of **SALT** and for **feeding support**. Isolated cleft lip babies can often still breastfeed or there are modified bottle teats available if there is palate involvement.
Surgical	• **Lip repair** usually around **3 months** of age. • **Palate repaired** at **6–12 months** of age (see *Fig. 3.18*). • Often need further **orthodontic surgery in later childhood**. • Long-term **ENT follow-up** as patients frequently have **otitis media** and Eustachian tube difficulties after surgical repair.
Psychosocial	• **Psychological support** for parents who may find their baby's appearance distressing. They should be **reassured that surgical outcomes are very good** and photos are useful to show what repairs look like postoperatively. • There are fantastic **support groups** that you can direct families; these include CLAPA (Cleft Lip and Palate Association) and Operation Smile.

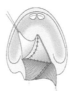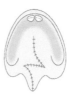

Fig. 3.18: Surgical technique for isolated cleft palate repair. This would be done at 6–12 months of age.

3.6.6 Spina bifida

Spina bifida is a term for a spectrum of types of neural tube defect (NTD), affecting 2–3:1000.

Pathophysiology

The brain and spinal cord develop from the **ectoderm-derived neural tube**. Spina bifida develops from **failure of the caudal end of the tube to close**. The neural tube closes **days 17–30 of gestation**.

Spina bifida is a spectrum of conditions; see *Table 3.15*.

Table 3.15: Types of spina bifida (see *Fig. 3.19*)		
Spina bifida occulta (SBO)	**Meningocele**	**Myelomeningocele**
• Vertebral arch defect with an **intact** spinal cord • Clinically apparent as a hairy patch of skin over the area • There is **no neurological deficit**	• Vertebral arch defect with herniation of the meninges but **not** the spinal cord • It is covered with skin • Prognosis following surgery is good, with <10% developing neurological impairment or hydrocephalus	• Thoracolumbar defect with herniation of the meninges **and spinal cord** • Only meninges covering neural tissue (no skin) • Prognosis depends on level and extent of lesion

Epidemiology and risk factors

Table 3.16: Risk factors for spina bifida	
Maternal folic acid deficiency	• Thought to be implicated in up to half of cases. Incidence has significantly decreased since the introduction of routine antenatal folic acid supplementation.
Maternal medications	• Anti-epileptics (especially valproate and carbamazepine).
Maternal diabetes	• Risk increases 2–10 fold.
Family history	• Risk increases to 1 in 20 with one previous child affected and to 1 in 2 if two previously affected.

Clinical features

Symptoms

- Depends on severity and spinal level.
- Myelomeningocele often causes hydrocephalus, bladder dysfunction and lower limb paralysis.

Signs

- Range from skin change (occulta) to bilateral lower limb paralysis and associated hydrocephalus (severe myelomeningocele).

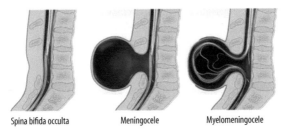

Spina bifida occulta   Meningocele   Myelomeningocele

Fig. 3.19: Types of spina bifida.

Investigation and diagnosis

Hx
- Often picked up on antenatal scans or with a raised **maternal alpha fetoprotein**.
- Ask about **family history** and if any **siblings** have an NTD.
- Is Mum **epileptic**, **diabetic**, or was the **pregnancy unplanned** (i.e. no folate)?
- Did Mum take folic acid supplements in early pregnancy?

Ex
- Birthweight, gestation, head size and shape.
- General appearance.
- Neurological exam – assess where the lowest level of motor and sensory function is. Where is the lesion and how extensive is it?
- Assess anal sphincter function and how the child is passing urine.
- Is there developmental dysplasia of the hip on examination? Talipes? Kyphoscoliosis?

Ix
- In high risk groups, **antenatal scans** by an experienced sonographer can identify NTDs and help prepare for treatment following delivery.
- **MRI scans** of brain and spinal cord for specific anatomy and to look for **Arnold–Chiari malformation** and evidence of **hydrocephalus**.
- **Lateral chest X-ray** to assess for scoliosis.

DDx
- Spina bifida occulta
- Meningocele
- Myelomeningocele
- Tethered spinal cord
- Spinal cord mass

Management

Medical

- For severe defects → **MDT management in a tertiary centre** (neurosurgeons, paediatricians, orthopaedics, urology, child development, psychology).
- Management of **neuropathic bladder** to minimize complications (such as UTI, reflux nephropathy leading to hypertension and chronic renal disease).

Surgical

- **Meningocele** and **myelomeningocele** are managed with surgical closure. With the lack of skin protection in the latter, surgery is undertaken as soon as possible to minimize infection risk.
- Close monitoring for development of **hydrocephalus** (and **VP (ventriculoperitoneal) shunt** insertion if needed).

Psychosocial

- Especially with the more severe defects these children will need lifelong complex care, which is a large burden on them and their families.
- **Specialist nurses** and early **psychological support** are very important factors.
- When discharged, GP and community paediatrics teams are imperative in ensuring good service coordination and quality of life for these families.

Chapter 4

Childhood growth

4.1 Failure to thrive

Failure to thrive (FTT) describes **inadequate weight gain** in an infant or young child. Defined as:

- children whose weight *crosses ≥2 centiles* on a growth chart or
- a child who is *persistently below the 5th percentile*.

Pathophysiology

An **organic cause will be found in <5%** of these children (see *Table 4.1*). The most **common pathophysiology is inadequate nutrition** ∴ the diagnostic question is: what is the cause of this?

Table 4.1: Pathophysiology of inadequate weight gain

Cause	Examples	Pathophysiology
Increased energy requirements	Congenital heart disease, cystic fibrosis, renal failure, immunodeficiency, malignancy, hyperthyroidism	Child cannot keep up with extra calorie intake needed to grow → growth falters
Inadequate absorption	Coeliac disease, short gut syndrome, cystic fibrosis, pancreatic insufficiency	Child cannot absorb enough nutrients to grow
Poor intake – physical	Reflux, neurological problem with impaired swallow, cleft palate, vomiting	Child physically cannot take sufficient nutrients
Poor intake – environmental	Inadequate food supply, poor socio-economic circumstances, maternal depression, poor parent–child interaction, neglect/abuse, fussy eating, behavioural difficulties	Child not being offered sufficient nutritional intake to reach their growth potential

Epidemiology and risk factors

Table 4.2: Risk factors for failure to thrive

Socio-economic deprivation	• Less money for food. Also associated with poorer parental education levels, so they may be less aware of nutritional requirements.
Chromosomal/genetic disorders	• Higher risk of neurological and gastrointestinal disorders, affecting ability to take and retain nutrition.
Maternal mental health issues	• Higher risk of Mum having poor interaction with the child, resulting in neglect.

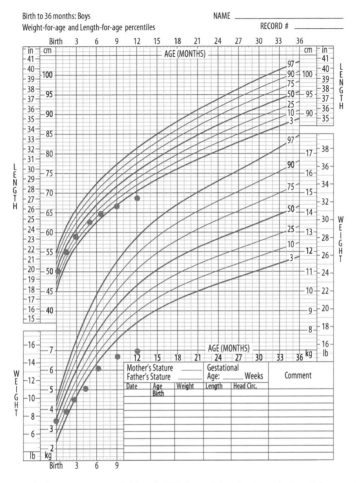

Fig. 4.1: A growth chart as seen in a child with FTT; the red dots indicate their weight crossing ≥2 centiles.

Investigation and diagnosis

Hx
- **Birthweight**, **gestation**, head size and shape. Birth **centiles**.
- Any psychological issues at home? Observe interaction between child and parents.
- Feeding history: what and how much is the child eating? Are meal times regular? What happens during meals?
- Family history of FTT including growth in siblings.
- History of medical issues, hospital admissions, prematurity.
- Symptoms suggestive of organic cause? (diarrhoea, cough, lethargy).

Ex
- **Developmental assessment** – is there evidence of delay or regression?
- **General appearance** – do they look well? Clean and kempt? Dysmorphic?
- **Cardiac exam** – evidence of cardiac failure? (hepatomegaly, breathlessness)
- **Respiratory** exam – clubbing? Chest deformity? Cough?
- **Abdominal** exam – peripheral signs of malabsorption? Distension? Buttock wasting?

Ix
- To identify if there is an organic cause (present in <5%).
- **Bloods** – **TFTs** (thyrotoxicosis), **FBC** (anaemia, malignancy), **U&Es** (renal failure, renal tubular acidosis), **CRP** (infection/inflammation), **coeliac screen**.
- **Stool sample** – infection, pancreatic insufficiency.
- **Urine sample** – renal disease, UTI.
- **CXR/sweat test** – cystic fibrosis.
- **Serial growth chart measurements** over time.

DDx
- Organic cause (listed under pathophysiology) or non-organic cause (environmental, neglect, abuse)

Management

- Most children can be **managed in primary care by increasing calorie intake** and monitoring response.
- Investigation is only needed if signs of organic cause are present or the child does not respond to increased calorie intake.
- **Social services** should be involved if there are concerns.
- **Dietitian** support is encouraged.
- **Speech and language therapists** if issue is feeding disorder.
- **Hospital admission is rarely indicated** → children usually respond very well once sufficient intake is established.

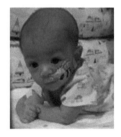

Fig. 4.2: A baby with FTT with an NG tube *in situ* to aid with feeding.

Short stature and poor growth

Short stature is defined as a child with **height <2nd centile**. This may be due to growth delay, familial short stature, organic reasons or constitutional short stature (2% of the population will fall naturally below the 2nd centile).

Pathophysiology

Growth is a complex interaction of hormones, genetics and environment. Your approach to the patient should aim to ascertain what the cause is.

Table 4.3: Pathophysiology of poor growth

Cause	Pathophysiology
Familial	Genetic potential means the child will be short.
Constitutional	Delay in puberty and thus growth. It is more common in boys. Growth tends to catch up to average height.
Growth hormone (GH) deficiency	Pituitary failure means body does not get signals to grow. This may be due to pituitary tumours, cranial radiation, pituitary trauma or an isolated endocrine growth hormone deficiency.
Hypothyroidism	Thyroid hormones are needed for normal GH secretion.
Corticosteroid excess	Has negative effect on bone formation, growth plate development and GH secretion → culminates in growth impairment at high enough doses. Often iatrogenic, but occasionally due to adrenal or pituitary pathology.
Nutritional	Insufficient calorie intake will result in growth impairment.
Chronic illness	Tend to be short **and** underweight. Chronic illness multifactorially has a negative impact on growth, both from endocrine perspective and due to increased calorie requirements.
Genetic	Many syndromes result in short stature. This may be proportional (Turner's syndrome, trisomy 21) or dysproportional (achondroplasia, other skeletal dysplasias).

Epidemiology and risk factors

Table 4.4: Risk factors for short stature	
Family history	• Most common cause. 1 in 50 children will fall below the 2nd centile. Working out **mid-parental height** (see *OSCE tips*) allows you to reassure family to absence of concerning pathology.
Poor nutritional intake	• Due to environment, chronic illness, deprivation or a combination. See *Section 4.1*. For poor intake to affect HEIGHT it must be **sustained** for a signifcant period of time (weight 1st → height 2nd → head circumference last).

Investigation and diagnosis

Hx
- Family history and close assessment of growth charts and growth velocity.
- History of steroid use? Visual changes (pituitary growths)? Chronic illness? FTT?

Ex
- Stature proportional (trunk and limbs in proportion) or disproportional?
- Dysmorphic features?
- Evidence on exam of underlying illness? Steroid excess (striae, Cushingoid facies)?
- How tall are the parents and siblings?
- Pubertal Tanner staging if old enough (*Fig. 2.1*).

Ix
- Growth charts including mid-parental height and growth velocity.
- **Bloods** (TFTs, insulin growth factor, CRP, U&Es)
- **Endocrine provocation / suppression tests** (GH deficiency, corticosteroid excess).
- **Imaging** – bone age (wrist X-ray). MRI brain if neurological features.

DDx
- See pathophysiology section. If in doubt seek an endocrinology opinion.

Management

- Depends on cause. Those with **constitutional** or **familial** short stature should be **reassured**.
- A paediatric endocrinologist should manage endocrine causes with the goal of achieving best possible adult height.
- **Growth hormone** is used to encourage growth in children with GH deficiency, Turner's syndrome, chronic renal failure and some IUGR patients.

OSCE tips: Calculating mid-parental height

A useful tool for assessing constitutional short stature and a child's genetic growth potential. Heights are measured in centimetres.

$$\text{Girl} = \frac{[\text{father's height} + \text{mother's height}] - 13}{2}$$

$$\text{Boy} = \frac{[\text{father's height} + \text{mother's height}] + 13}{2}$$

Normal range is ± 10 cm

Chapter 5

Child abuse

> "If you don't think, you won't diagnose."
> From the *Child Protection Companion*, published by the RCPCH.

Introduction

Child abuse can be defined as **'any act of commission or omission which results in harm to the child'**,[1] and the ability to recognise children who are victims of abuse, as well as knowing the actions to take in these instances, is a **core skill** of *all* doctors. Early identification is essential and will make an enormous difference to the child, allowing them to access the care and support that they require.

As a junior doctor your responsibility will not be to make definitive decisions about the abused child, but to recognise the signs and know the next steps to take. You will almost certainly see suspected or confirmed cases of child abuse during your paediatrics training.

Identifying at-risk children

The General Medical Council (GMC) provides some key points to be aware of in identifying at-risk children or young people:

- Be aware of risk factors that have been linked to abuse and neglect and look out for signs that a child or young person may be at risk (see *Section 5.3*).
- If you are treating an adult patient, consider whether your patient poses a risk to children or young people.
- Keep an open mind and be objective when making decisions. Work in partnership with families where possible.
- If you are not sure about whether a child or young person is at risk or how best to act on your concerns, ask a named or designated professional or a lead clinician or, if they are not available, an experienced colleague for advice.

The GMC's publication, *Protecting Children and Young People*, is an excellent resource that outlines the key duties and responsibilities of a doctor in safeguarding children.

---

[1] RCPCH *Child Protection Companion*. Available at www.rcpch.ac.uk

Physical abuse

Encompassing **any behaviour which is injurious or causes physical harm to the child**, this term also includes those cases where a parent or carer fabricates (or deliberately induces) illness in a child – termed 'fabricated or induced injury' (FII, previously 'Munchausen syndrome by proxy').

5.2.1 History

- **Vague or inconsistent** stories which may not make sense, or fail to explain the injury adequately.
- The mode of injury may have been '**unwitnessed**'.
- There may have been a **time delay** between the injury and presentation.
- Is the child immobile? **Infants who cannot move** rarely have accidental injuries.
- Presence of **multiple injuries** is suspicious.

5.2.2 Bruises

- No specific bruise is pathognomic, but there are characteristics that should raise suspicion. **Accidental bruises are found in mobile children, usually over bony prominences or on the shin**.
- Sites of non-accidental bruising are illustrated in *Fig. 5.1*.
- Type:
  - Look for patterns consistent with a **slap mark or implements**, such as belts or sticks (see *Fig. 5.2*).
  - Bruises that are **clustered** or **contain petechiae** are of concern.

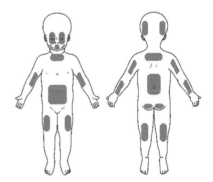

Fig. 5.1: Sites of non-accidental bruising: head, ear, mastoid process, eyes, mouth, mandible, neck, chest, abdomen, lower back and buttocks.

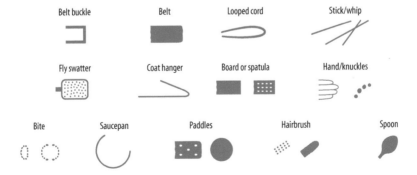

Fig. 5.2: Patterns left by commonly used implements in physical abuse of children.

> **OSCE tips 1:** Clotting disorder
>
> **Clotting disorder should always be considered as a differential,** so ensure you take a full personal and family history of coagulopathy.

5.2.3 Bites

- Bite marks are usually easily identified; however, one needs to decide if the bite is from an **animal or a human and, if human, an adult or child.**

Human bite

- **Human bites are 'U-shaped'** and, since the incisors and canines are of similar length, all of these teeth may leave a mark. It's not uncommon for both the upper and lower teeth to mark the skin, giving a **circular appearance**.
- The distinction between adult and child bite is difficult, so contact the **forensic odontologist** and take a **skin swab** to aid DNA identification.

Animal (dog) bite

- Animal bites are usually from a dog. Characteristically, they have **four prominent, sharp canines** that puncture the skin and a **'V-shaped' dental arch**.

5.2.4 Fractures

- 80% of non-accidental fractures occur in children under 18 months of age.

Table 5.1: Fractures that should raise the suspicion of abuse	
Skull	<ul><li>Commonest: linear parietal fracture</li><li>Complex or multiple fracture ± crossing the suture line</li><li>Wide fracture</li><li>Occipital fracture (requires very high force)</li></ul>
Spine	<ul><li>Frequently accompanied by head injury</li><li>Cervical spine – occurs in a shaken baby</li><li>Thoracolumbar fracture</li><li>Compression fracture</li></ul>
Thorax	<ul><li>Rib fractures, particularly in very young infants (shaken baby)</li><li>Posterior rib fractures are more common in abused children</li></ul>
Upper limb	<ul><li>Spiral fracture of the humerus is strongly linked with abuse</li></ul>
Lower limb	<ul><li>Femoral fractures of any type, in immobile children only</li></ul>
Metaphyseal fracture	<ul><li>Unusual fractures, particularly before 2 years of age</li><li>Femoral metaphyseal fractures are strongly linked with abuse</li></ul>

OSCE tips 2: DDx for childhood fractures

There are a number of differential diagnoses for fractures in children. In the neonatal period, **obstetric trauma** may be the cause. Later, consider **osteogenesis imperfecta, osteopenia, infection / osteomyelitis and malignancy**.

5.2.5 Non-accidental head injury

- Non-accidental head injury (NAHI) was previously called 'shaken baby'.
- Under the age of 1 year, 95% of head injuries are non-accidental. Of these patients, **≤30% will die and ~50% have residual neurodisability** (of varying degree).
- Due to severe, **repetitive rotational injury and/or a direct head impact** that may result in a **constellation** of different injuries:

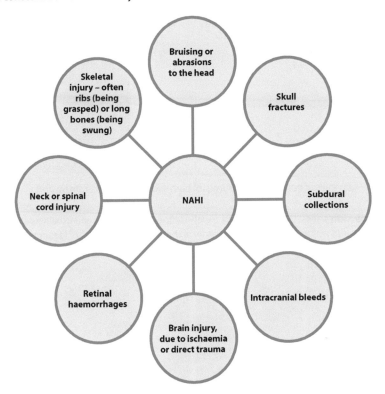

Fig. 5.3: Injuries that may result from NAHI.

- As any number of the injuries shown in *Fig. 5.3* can be sustained, the **presentation of these patients is variable**, ranging from **poor feeding and lethargy, to seizures, respiratory depression and sudden death**.
- *In all cases where this is suspected, ensure you examine the fundus with a direct ophthalmoscope.* Characteristically, **retinal haemorrhages** are seen.

5.2.6 Intra-abdominal injury

- Any viscera may be injured, but the **small bowel** is particularly common.
- Presentation can vary, from unexplained collapse to sepsis and abdominal pain.

5.2.7 Thermal injury

- Burns and scalds are especially common in children and in many cases the cause is accidental. Despite this, it is important to always consider non-accidental injury (or neglectful parenting) in these children.
- Sites: most often the **hands**, **feet**, **buttocks**, **legs** and **face**.
- Characteristic non-accidental burns:
  - **Contact** burns (e.g. cooker hotplate, iron): **well-defined** outlines resembling the implement.

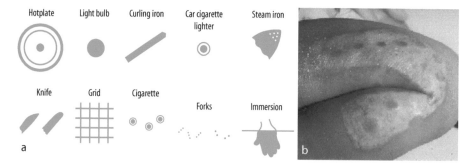

Fig. 5.4: (a) examples of non-accidental burns; (b) burn showing outline of steam iron.

  - **Immersion** scalds: these burns have a **well-defined upper limit** and usually *spare the surface that was pressed against the bottom of the bath* (i.e. pale soles of feet or buttocks).

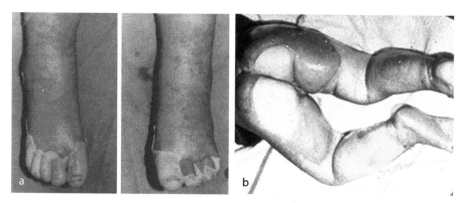

Fig. 5.5: (a) immersion scald; (b) spared surface.

- In accidental burns the child will often flail, producing **splash marks**; these are usually **absent** in non-accidental injuries.

Other burn types:

- Scalds from **thrown hot liquid**: no defining features.
- **Friction** burns: from being dragged along the floor.
  - In such instances, look in the mouth, as there may be a **torn upper labial frenulum**.

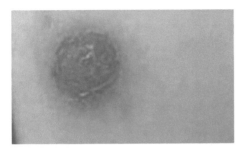

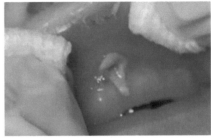

Fig. 5.6: Cigarette burns: appropriately sized with a deep, cratered appearance and ulcerated centre.

Fig. 5.7: Torn upper labial frenulum, characteristic of friction burn.

Investigations

A number of investigations may be relevant depending on the presentation of the child, so perform only those that are pertinent:

- **Photograph** all injuries and include a **ruler** (with mm denominations) in the **image**.
- **Swabs** of skin if bite mark.
- **Urinalysis** if abdominal trauma is suspected, as this may reveal **haematuria**.
- Bloods:
  - if bruising – to identify **coagulopathy**:
    - film
    - FBC and WCC
    - clotting
  - if a fracture – to identify **organic bone disease**:
    - consider Ca^{2+}, phosphate, ALP, vitamin D
  - if abdominal injury suspected:
    - serial FBC – for blood loss
    - amylase – pancreatic or splenic injury
    - LFTs – transiently elevated in hepatic trauma
- Plain film **X-ray** if fracture suspected
- **CT head ± MRI in NAHI is essential**
- Others:
  - **skeletal survey** – a **series** of radiographs that systematically cover the **entire skeleton**, indicated in children with **suspected non-accidental fractures or NAHI**; this may be repeated after 11–14 days
  - bone scan
  - septic screen – to exclude infection (for example, in a drowsy baby).

Emotional abuse

Emotional abuse is the persistent **behaviours of the child's carer** towards them, which include **criticism**, **denigration** (to speak ill of or belittle), **rejection and 'scapegoating'**. It is difficult to detect as it may present with a wide array of different, **non-specific symptoms** (*Table 5.2*), but it is *usually found in association with other forms of abuse*.

Table 5.2: Symptoms of emotional abuse in different age groups	
Younger child	• Failure to thrive • Developmental delay (particularly language and social skills) • Poor sleep pattern • Other behaviours on spectrum and non-specific
Older child	• Poor school performance or truancy • Wetting and soiling • Feelings of worthlessness, inadequacy and isolation
Adolescent	• Confrontational, aggressive and delinquent behaviours • Acts of self-harm and substance abuse • May develop depression or eating disorders

An awareness of the risk factors for child abuse is key to helping identify children who are at risk of abuse and neglect. They can be broadly categorized into three groups (*Table 5.3*):

Table 5.3: Risk factors for child abuse	
Parental factors	• Parent suffered abuse as a child themselves • Parent has a mental illness • Parent abuses drugs or alcohol • Parent is unsupported • Parent is young with a low level of education • Parent has poor knowledge of parenting and unrealistic expectations of the child
Environmental factors	• Family violence • Poverty • High rates of disadvantage in their community • Overcrowding • Multiple family stressors
Child factors	• The child/pregnancy was unwanted • The child has a disability and needs a high degree of care • Child falls ill before the age of 6 months

Neglect

Neglect is the 'persistent failure to meet a child's basic physical and/or psychological needs, likely to result in the serious impairment of the child's health or development'.[2] In accordance with the definition it is largely a **chronic** behaviour, but may be episodic in some instances, especially when there is a family crisis. Neglect can take many forms including the **failure to meet the child's physical**, **hygiene**, **medical**, **supervision**, **stimulation**, **social** or **affection needs**.

Presentation of neglect	
Physical and hygiene	• The **cleanliness and appearance** of the child is unacceptable, and they may **be inappropriately dressed** for the occasion/season. • **Failure to thrive** due to inappropriate diet.
Medical	• **Poor uptake of immunizations** and untreated or **inadequately cared for medical conditions**. It is important to recognize that disabled children are very vulnerable to neglect and so these medical conditions may be very severe in some instances.
Supervision	• **Recurrent A&E attendances** for accidental injury.
Stimulation	• **Developmental delay** and poor school performance.
Social	• **Challenging** behaviours.

OSCE tips 3: A systematic approach to a child protection station

- Identify risk factors: parental, environmental and child factors.
- History of presenting complaint (HPC): vague / inconsistent, unwitnessed or time delay to presentation?
- Past medical history (PMH): recurrent admissions? Up to date with immunizations? If they have previous co-morbidities, are they adequately cared for?
- Development: reaching developmental milestones at the correct times?
- Examination: general appearance? Are they failing to thrive?
  - systematic examination that includes looking at the fundi
- Investigations: basic investigations but do not undertake any 'forensic' assessments.
- Management:
  - early senior involvement and escalation
  - accurate documentation and photographs if possible
  - refer to the appropriate authorities – gain consent to do so
  - assess the need for admission of the child.

---

[2] HM Government, 2018. *Working Together to Safeguard Children*. Available at bit.ly/WTSC2018.

Sexual abuse

Whilst of serious concern in its own right, sexual abuse is very commonly associated with other forms of abuse, underlining further the importance of its recognition. Where there is suspicion, the junior doctor **should immediately enlist the help of their seniors**.

Presentation

There are no pathognomic signs for sexual abuse per se, but there are symptoms and signs that should raise concerns:

Genital features	Behavioural features
• Vaginal bleeding • Rectal bleeding • Vulvovaginitis • Anogenital warts • Pregnancy, the presence of semen and sexually transmitted infections are all relatively strong indicators of sexual abuse in children • Foreign body in vagina or anus	• Excessive masturbation that is done in public, or interferes with life • Soiling, encopresis or enuresis • A major change in the child's behaviour

5.6 Fabricated or induced illness (FII)

Fabricated or induced illness (previously 'Munchausen syndrome by proxy') is the current term used to describe this form of abuse, as, unlike its predecessor, it does not place the onus of blame on the child; the perpetrator in most instances is the **parent or primary caregiver**. The spectrum of symptoms in these children is **very wide**, ranging from trivial injuries to death, but they **share common features**, as shown in *Fig. 5.8*.

The child presents **recurrently** with symptoms that **warrant multiple procedures**

The perpetrator **cannot give any aetiological factors** for the child's illness

The symptoms described by the perpetrator **do not fit with those that are observed by the medical team**

The child's symptoms and signs may **regress or disappear with removal of the perpetrator**

Fig. 5.8: Features of FII.

Management of child abuse is discussed in general in *Section 5.7*; however, it is important to note that *in cases of suspected FII, the assumed perpetrator is not informed of your concerns*.

Management

As a junior doctor, it will **not** be your responsibility to perform detailed examinations, investigations and management of these children. Rather, one should aim to *identify the cases in a timely manner* and **undertake the** *basic initial* **management**.

- Contact your **senior** and/or the **lead paediatrician in child protection**.
  - **Gather information** from other professionals who know the child.
  - **Check** if the child is on the **child protection register**.
- *Document everything carefully, precisely and extensively*.
- Take **photographs** if appropriate.
- Initiate some **basic investigations**.

> Over 48 000 children in England were identified as needing protection from abuse in 2017

What to tell the parents?

- In general, the parents **are** informed of what is happening, *as is the child*; however, **do not accuse anybody** of harming the child.
  - The exceptions to this principle (that is, when you do not tell the parents) are when:
    - you consider that telling the parents would **put the child or their siblings at risk of harm**
    - **fabricated or induced illness (FII) is suspected**.

Who to refer to?

Social services	Police

• This is the central agency to which **all cases of suspected (or confirmed) abuse or neglect should be referred**. This is done over the telephone on the same day and confirmed via letter within 48 hours.
• If the child or sibling is at risk of **further harm**, or **serious abuse was witnessed**, an **immediate** referral should be made.
	• The police deal with criminal acts or where extra powers of protection are needed.
	• A referral is needed if:
	  • Allegations of **rape/sexual abuse**.
	  • Severely injured or dead child where **abuse is suspected**.
	  • The perpetrator is **threatening to remove the child** from hospital where the child is thought to be in immediate danger.

Where does the child go?

In most instances, the child is not admitted to hospital and can go home, having had the **appropriate medical management and the required referrals made**. It is the children's social services that will then follow up and investigate the suspected cases of abuse.

Chapter 6

The febrile child

Introduction

The febrile child (T >38°C) is one of the most common reasons for medical attention. As with many childhood presentations the diagnosis is often benign, but **may be life-threatening**. In this chapter we discuss how to **assess** and **investigate** children with different types of fever: 'acute' and 'pyrexia of unknown origin (PUO)'. The individual diagnoses are discussed elsewhere in the book.

There is an important distinction to be made regarding 'acute fever' vs. PUO:

- Acute fever: a short history of illness
- PUO: a single illness lasting ≥**3 weeks** with a fever present most days, and **no diagnosis after 1 week of inpatient investigation.**

6.1 Acute fever

Accounting for ~20% of emergency department (ED) visits, these children present with a short history of fever. They often have an infection and require **urgent investigation ± empirical treatment**. A comprehensive, **structured** evaluation is very important; however, it is essential to recognize that **children <3 y/o may only have vague symptoms and signs**. After this age, symptoms and signs in children are generally more readily identifiable.

Pathophysiology

The differential diagnosis can be considered using a systems-based approach:

Body system	Differential diagnosis
Central nervous system (CNS)	Meningitis Encephalitis Cerebral abscess
Ears	Otitis media
Nose	Sinusitis
Throat	Upper respiratory tract infection (URTI) Quinsy Epiglottitis
Neck	Meningitis / encephalitis
Respiratory	Pneumonia Croup Bronchiolitis
Cardiac	Infective endocarditis Myocarditis
Gastrointestinal	Gastroenteritis Meckel diverticulum Mesenteric adenitis Appendicitis
Hepatobiliary	Hepatitis Pancreatitis Cholecystitis
Genitourinary	Pyelonephritis UTI
Musculoskeletal	Septic arthritis Osteomyelitis

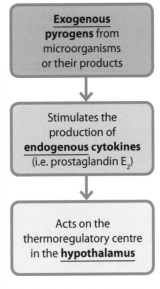

Fig 6.1: Basic pathophysiology of acute fever.

Clinical features

The first assessment to be made is the **seriousness of the illness**. This can done using a 'traffic light' system, as described by NICE (2013) CG160:

	Green – low risk	Amber – intermediate risk	Red – high risk
Colour (of skin, lips or tongue)	• Normal colour	• Pallor reported by parent / carer	• Pale/mottled/ashen/blue
Activity	• Responds normally to social cues • Content/smiles • Stays awake or awakens quickly • Strong normal cry/ not crying	• Not responding normally to social cues • No smile • Wakes only with prolonged stimulation • Decreased activity	• No response to social cues • Appears ill to a healthcare professional • Does not wake or if roused does not stay awake • Weak, high-pitched or continuous cry

Respiratory		• Nasal flaring
		• Tachypnoea:
		  • RR >50 breaths/minute, age 6–12 months
		  • RR >40 breaths/minute, age >12 months
		• Oxygen saturation ≤95% in air
		• Crackles in the chest
			• Grunting
			• Tachypnoea: RR >60 breaths/minute
			• Moderate or severe chest indrawing

Circulation and hydration	• Normal skin and eyes
	• Moist mucous membranes
		• Tachycardia:
		  • >160 beats/minute, age <12 months
		  • >150 beats/minute, age 12–24 months
		  • >140 beats/minute, age 2–5 years
		• CRT ≥3 seconds
		• Dry mucous membranes
		• Poor feeding in infants
		• Reduced urine output
			• Reduced skin turgor

Other	• None of the amber or red symptoms or signs	• Age 3–6 months, temperature ≥39°C • Fever for ≥5 days • Rigors • Swelling of a limb or joint • Non-weight bearing limb/ not using an extremity	• Age <3 months, temperature ≥38°C* • Non-blanching rash • Bulging fontanelle • Neck stiffness • Status epilepticus • Focal neurological signs • Focal seizures

Fig 6.2: Traffic light system for identifying risk of serious illness.
*Some vaccinations have been found to induce fever in children aged under 3 months.

OSCE tips: Measurement of temperature in children

It is recommended that temperature is measured either via the (a) tympanic membrane or (b) axilla. Oral and rectal measurements are not recommended.

Clinical features

Hx

HPC:
- Characterize the fever: onset, height, duration and fluctuance.
- Is there are rash? These are common in children. ?Non-blanching (→ septicaemia)

Systems review:
- A structured interrogation of **all the major organ systems** (→ refer to *Section 1.1* for information).

Birth, Feeding, Immunization and Development (BiFID):
- Recent immunization? This is a cause of fever.
- Lack of immunization predisposes to bacterial infection.

PMH:
- Conditions predisposing to infection (e.g. sickle cell disease, congenital heart disease, HIV)

DH:
- Newly introduced medication (especially those with anticholinergic effects).

SH:
- Recent travel? (→ mosquitoes? TB?)
- Exposure to unwell contacts?

Ex
- Baseline observations
- Assessment of hydration status
- Rashes?
- Lymphadenopathy?
- A structured assessment of **all the major organ systems**, including ENT

Ix

These vary depending on the child's age and the seriousness of the illness (→ colour on the 'traffic light' system); children >3 months old with 'green' examination findings **do not routinely need investigation**. Investigations should be **targeted** towards the likely diagnosis; however, in the absence of a clear source of infection, a generic approach is taken. This is presented below:

Bloods:
- FBC, CRP, blood cultures and blood gas

Urine dip:
- All children, including the 'green' group

Lumbar puncture:
- All children <3 months, or

- Any age with 'red' signs, or
- <1 year and 'amber'

CXR:
- If respiratory symptoms present or
- If 'red' or 'amber' signs

Management

Table 6.1: Management of acute fever	
Definitive	• Antibiotics: ideally **after** specimens are collected • Consider admission to hospital if 'amber' or 'red': if the clinical condition warrants it or there are social circumstances necessitating it (including ↑ parental anxiety)
Symptomatic	• Antipyretics: used if the child is distressed only – they are not to be used if the only intention is reducing a fever (when the child is not distressed by it)

Safety-netting	Adequate parental 'safety-netting' advice:
	• When to return to hospital:
	  • >5 days duration
	  • non-blanching rash develops
	  • seizure
	  • symptoms deteriorate
	  • parents unable to cope
	• Child to stay away from school whilst unwell
	• Encourage ↑ oral intake at home

Rapid diagnosis – recognition of sepsis in children

If signs of shock or sepsis → ABCDE, empirical antibiotics and IV fluids. Refer to critical care.

There is extensive guidance available for the recognition and treatment of sepsis, and we advise that you refer to national and local guidelines. The broad features assessed are as follows:
- Behaviour: altered Glasgow Coma Scale (GCS), weak cry, decreased activity
- Appearance: mottled / ashen / cyanosed / non-blanching rash
- Cardiac: tachycardia (or <60 bpm). Delayed capillary refill time
- Respiratory: tachypnoea (or apnoea / grunting)
- Genitourinary: reduced urine output
- Lactate: >2mmol/L

Pyrexia of unknown origin (PUO)

Pyrexia of unknown origin (PUO) is a single illness lasting ≥**3 weeks** with a fever present most days, and **no diagnosis after 1 week of inpatient investigation**. The three most common groups of diagnoses are **infection**, **connective tissue disorder** and **neoplasm** (see *Fig. 6.3*).

Pathophysiology

PUO is <u>most often</u> a **common condition presenting in an unusual way** and, therefore, all of the diagnoses stated in *Section 6.1* are also important differentials.

The additional diagnoses that should also be considered include:

Infectious	Kawasaki disease, TB, typhoid fever, cat-scratch disease (*Bartonella henselae*), malaria, infectious mononucleosis, HIV
Connective tissue disorders	Juvenile idiopathic arthritis (JIA), systemic lupus erythematosus (SLE), sarcoidosis
Inflammatory	Ulcerative colitis (UC), Crohn's disease
Neoplastic	(Hodgkin) lymphoma, leukaemia
Endocrine	Hyperthyroidism
Other	Factitious disorders or FII

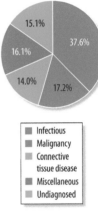

Fig 6.3: The most common groups of diagnoses in children with PUO.

Investigation and diagnosis

Ix

- Bloods: FBC, ESR, CRP, blood cultures, ± renal profile, ± liver profile, ± thyroid function tests
- Consider **disease-specific** blood tests:
  - HIV/EBV/CMV serology
  - TB serology
  - ANA/dsDNA/C3/C4 (→ ?SLE)
- Nasopharyngeal swab (→ ?viruses)
- Urine dip
- Stool culture
- Lumbar puncture
- CXR
- Echocardiogram (→ ?infective endocarditis)
- Further imaging: such as USS or CT/MRI
- ± Bone marrow aspirate (→ ?lymphoma/leukaemia)
- ± Biopsies (i.e. of skin lesions, lymph nodes or masses)

Management

- Unlike in acute fever, empirical treatment for PUO is **not** advocated.
- Repeated clinical examination.
- Symptomatic treatment.
- Definitive management is treatment of the underlying diagnosis.

Chapter 7

Childhood allergy

Allergic rhinitis

Allergic rhinitis ('**hay fever**') is inflammation of the nasal epithelium in response to an allergen, which results in characteristic sneezing, coughing, rhinorrhoea and red itchy eyes.

Pathophysiology

Multifactorial predisposition, partially genetic and partially environmental. The final common pathway is **abnormal IgE-mediated immune response** to an allergen (typically grasses, pollens, pets, dust mites) → known as a **type 1 hypersensitivity reaction**.

- **Early phase** (*Fig. 7.1*)– IgE-mediated **mast cell degranulation** releases **histamine** directly, causing allergic effects (sneezing, urticaria or angioedema and bronchospasm in anaphylaxis).
- **Late phase** – 4–6 hours later **eosinophils, basophils** and **T cells** release mediators that cause **nasal inflammation** resulting in congestion and rhinorrhoea.

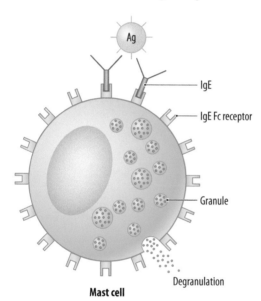

Ag

IgE

IgE Fc receptor

Granule

Degranulation

Mast cell

Fig 7.1: The early phase reaction in allergic rhinitis. An allergen binds to IgE receptors on the surface of mast cells → triggering degranulation and **histamine** release.

Epidemiology and risk factors

- Population prevalence 20–40%.
- Higher in those with a strong family history of atopy (eczema, hay fever or asthma).

Table 7.1: Risk factors for allergic rhinitis	
Family history	• Especially for hay fever/asthma/eczema, a family history of atopy will be present in most cases
Presence of other atopy	• Mediated by same mechanism so presence of one allergic condition makes another far more likely

Investigation and diagnosis

Hx   **Sneezing/rhinorrhoea/red itchy eyes**. Ask about family history, seasonal variance and if a trigger is identifiable.

Ex   Look for **eczema**, examine chest for signs of **asthma**, look for **nasal polyps** and oedema/inflammation. **Postnasal drip** may produce a **chronic dry cough**.

DDx
- Choanal atresia
- Rhinosinusitis
- Nasal foreign body
- Nasal polyps

Management

1. Limit allergen exposure.
2. Non-sedating **antihistamines** (loratidine, fexofenadine).
3. **Sodium cromoglycate** eye drops.
4. Severe cases may require systemic leukotriene receptor antagonists (**montelukast**).
5. Management of other atopic conditions if present (asthma, eczema).

7.2 Food allergy

Pathophysiology

- **IgE-mediated.** The mast cell degranulation in food allergy acts systemically to produce a range of symptoms from urticaria (mild) to angioedema and bronchospasm (severe) → characteristic of **anaphylactic** reaction.
- Allergy may be **primary** (the child has never developed immune tolerance to substance) or **secondary** (child previously tolerated substance but has developed cross-sensitivity intolerance to it). **Secondary allergies tend to be less severe.**

Epidemiology and risk factors

Seen in **6% of children**, most commonly to nuts, milk, eggs, seafood, seeds and fruits. Falls to **2% by adulthood**.

Table 7.2: Risk factors for food allergy	
Family history	• Less so than in atopic conditions but still increases risk
Non-breastfed infant	• Breastfeeding up to 6 months reduces rate of food allergy

Investigation and diagnosis

Hx
- Onset of symptoms 10–15 minutes after food ingestion.
- Typically, urticaria and a rash.
- In anaphylaxis → angioedema of the eye/mouth/face, voice change, sensation of tight chest and cough/wheeze. **Stridor** develops as the airway closes from **laryngeal oedema**.

Ix
Skin prick testing (*Fig. 7.2*) – multiple potential allergens are put on skin with control substance (histamine). Areas that redden suggest IgE-mediated allergy to that substance.

DDx
Food intolerance – presents with diarrhoea/vomiting or abdominal pain/colic. Non-IgE-mediated.

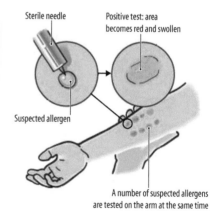

Sterile needle

Positive test: area becomes red and swollen

Suspected allergen

A number of suspected allergens are tested on the arm at the same time

Fig 7.2: Skin prick testing.

Management

> **ANAPHYLAXIS**
>
> 1. **ABCDE.** High-flow **oxygen**.
> 2. **IM adrenaline 1:1000**. (0.15ml up to 6 yrs, 0.3ml 6–12 yrs, 0.5ml >12 yrs). Repeat as needed.
> 3. **20ml/kg IV fluid bolus**.
> 4. IV **hydrocortisone**.
> 5. IV **chlorphenamine**.
> 6. **Salbutamol** nebulizers for bronchospasm.

Long term

- **Education** on avoiding offending allergens.
- **EpiPen** and education on use.
- **Dietitian** input if multiple allergies/failure to thrive.
- **Testing to identify other allergens** may be indicated in difficult-to-diagnose cases.

Chapter 8

Respiratory disorders

Upper respiratory tract infections

Upper respiratory tract infections (URTIs) are responsible for a **significant number of consultations and missed school days**. The term URTI recognizes that the infection may lie anywhere along the course of the upper respiratory tract (see *Fig. 8.1*); however, the exact site is not often explicitly known – indeed, many of these structures are often involved concurrently in a child.

Pathophysiology

- **Most URTIs are viral** in origin: typically, rhinovirus or coronavirus.

- Inoculation may occur:

  - if a child touches their nose or mouth following **direct contact with an infected surface**

  - via the **inhalation of respiratory droplets** from an infected person.

- Viruses then **invade the mucosal surface**, producing an **inflammatory response**.

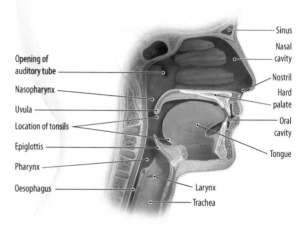

Fig. 8.1: Structures of the upper respiratory tract.

Epidemiology and risk factors

- URTIs are the **most common infectious illness** in children.

Table 8.1: Risk factors for URTI	
School attendance	• Children are in close contact with a large reservoir of infectious agents.
Second-hand smoking	• Can damage mucosa leading to increased susceptibility.
Immunocompromised state	• Such as those with congenital immunodeficiencies.

Clinical features

Symptoms

- The leading symptoms tend to be **mild and non-specific**, and include:
  - nasal obstruction and sneezing
  - nasal discharge (often clear)
  - a sore throat
  - a headache.

- A **cough** is found in about one-third of patients and is non-productive.
- The child may be **febrile**. This is more pronounced in infants and may be the presenting symptom in this group.
- Particularly in very young children, **feeding** may be affected.

Signs

- It should be noted that **the heterogeneity of this condition means that signs may be present or absent**, and found in various combinations.
- A thorough **respiratory and ENT assessment** are required, as well as the child's **hydration status and growth** if they are not feeding well.
- Baseline observations: the child may be **febrile**, but other observations are usually normal.

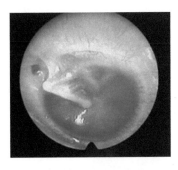

Fig. 8.2: Otitis media with effusion.

- Respiratory:
    - often nil.
- ENT:
    - ears: **otitis media with effusion** may be seen (the tympanic membranes appear dull, grey-yellow in colour and retracted – *Fig. 8.2*)
    - nose: the nasal mucosa may be **erythematous and discharge** may be visible
    - throat: **pharyngeal erythema and tonsillar swelling** may be present (*Fig. 8.3*).

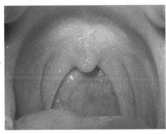

Fig. 8.3: Pharyngeal erythema.

OSCE tips 1: ENT examination in children	
	• Generally, ENT assessment should be done at the end of your examination, as it will often cause distress to the child. Demonstrating on their parents first may help.
Ears	Remember that the ear is pulled anteriorly and inferiorly in children, and do not forget to inspect the mastoid process.
Nose	Lift the tip of the nose gently and, using the largest attachment of the *auroscope*, gently place the tip inside the naris. Look **posteriorly**, rather than superiorly.
Throat	This is the most unpleasant part for young children and can be technically the most challenging for two reasons: • The child will not open their mouth. • The pharynx cannot be easily visualized. In these cases, you should try to insert the tongue depressor as it is a necessary part of the examination. If this upsets the patient and they start crying, **be savvy**: use this as an opportunity to visualize the pharynx.

Investigation and diagnosis

Hx
- A variety of vague symptoms attributable to the URT.
- A paucity of other localizing respiratory symptoms.
- The child may be febrile and off food.

Ex
- The chest is clear on examination.
- ENT examination should seek to identify the source.

Ix
- Generally, a clinical diagnosis.
- If persistent, swabs can be taken for microscopy, culture and sensitivity.

DDx
- Allergic rhinitis
- Infectious mononucleosis (teenagers)
- Asthma
- Pneumonia
- Otitis media

Management

- Management is **conservative** and symptomatic.
- Non-pharmacogical:
  - encourage good **oral hydration** and food intake.
  - **inhalation of steam** may be of benefit (run a warm shower and sit with the child in the bathroom).
- Pharmacological:
  - simple analgesics and anti-pyretics such as **paracetamol and ibuprofen.**
  - over-the-counter **cough syrups** may be of benefit.
  - antibiotics are **not** indicated in URTIs, unless prolonged and/or suspected bacterial infections.

Clinical pharmacology – Paracetamol and ibuprofen prescribing in children

Paracetamol and ibuprofen should **not** be taken at the same time in children, in order to avoid administration mistakes and therefore toxicity.

Begin with paracetamol as required and, if this is not sufficient, switch to ibuprofen. Where this proves ineffective, alternate administration of both medications and ask the parents to start a treatment diary.

8.2 Epiglottitis

Epiglottitis is acute inflammation of the epiglottis that can lead to serious airway obstruction. Following *Haemophilus influenzae type B* (HIB) vaccination, epiglottitis is now **uncommon**; however, children still die from this condition and **a high degree of clinical suspicion is required**.

Pathophysiology

- Epiglottitis is usually a bacterial infection caused by **HIB**, *Pneumococcus*, **Group A beta-haemolytic streptococci** and *Pseudomonas*.
  - viruses (HSV), fungi (*Candida albicans*) and traumatic insults, such as heat or chemical injury, may also be causal.
- The epiglottis and its surrounding tissues become **acutely** inflamed. This leads to **pharyngeal obstruction** which is a **surgical emergency**.

Epidemiology and risk factors

- Epiglottitis accounts for approximately 600 admissions in England annually.
- **Most commonly seen before 8 years of age**, although it may occur at **any** age.

Table 8.2: Major risk factors for epiglottitis	
Non-vaccination	• Although vaccination does not entirely preclude this possibility.
Immunocompromise	• Predisposes to epiglottitis and its more severe forms.

Clinical features

Symptoms (The 4 Ds)
- Early: **D**rooling and **D**ysphagia/Odynophagia
- Late: **D**ysphonia and **D**yspnoea
- Rapidly progressing sore throat (hours) should prompt consideration of this diagnosis.

Signs
- The patient **looks unwell**.
- Children may adopt the **'tripod' position** (*Fig. 8.4*).
- Baseline observations show a **high temperature**.
- General examination may elicit **cervical lymphadenopathy**.
- Respiratory examination:
  - **respiratory distress:** nasal flaring, tracheal tug, raising the shoulders, intercostal recession
  - an inspiratory *stridor is a late sign, and indicates upper airway narrowing*.

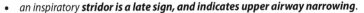

Fig. 8.4: The 'tripod' position. The child leans forward with both arms outstretched and their tongue out.

Investigations and diagnosis

- As epiglottitis is an emergency, diagnosis is often based on history and examination only.

Hx
- Vaccination history.
- Ask about the onset (rapidly progressing sore throat) and the 4 Ds.

Ex
- Look for tripod position, respiratory distress, stridor and fever.

Ix
- **Laryngoscopy: gold standard** and should be performed in an area that has access to an emergency airway.
  - rarely, an X-ray of the lateral cervical neck may be done which will show an enlarged, swollen epiglottis – the 'thumbprint sign'.
- **Swabs**: from the throat for MC&S.
- **Bloods:**
  - culture
  - blood gases (if septic – raised lactate and a metabolic acidosis)
  - FBC, CRP, U&E (confirm infective cause)

DDx
- Peritonsillar abscess ('quinsy')
- Tonsillitis
- Retropharyngeal abscess
- Laryngotracheobronchitis
- Aspirated foreign body

Management

- Patients will generally be managed on the **intensive care unit** (*Table 8.3*).

Table 8.3: Principles of epiglottitis management

Initially, secure the airway	• Give **high flow oxygen** through a non-rebreather mask • If tolerated, **nebulized adrenaline** can afford temporary improvement • **Intubation is first line** for airway management and is usually done at laryngoscopy
Treat the infection	• IV **antibiotics**, according to local guidelines
Provide therapeutic adjuncts	• IV **steroid**, to reduce inflammation • IV **maintenance fluids** as the patient is nil by mouth
Recovery	• Extubation is usually performed at around 72 hours, after which antibiotic treatment is switched to an oral preparation

Management of child with epiglottitis	
DO:	DO NOT:
• Call for senior help and get the crash trolley. • Contact senior ENT and anaesthetic doctors, and ask for their help. • Keep the child calm.	• Attempt direct examination of the pharynx using a tongue depressor if epiglottitis is suspected. These patients are at risk of reflex laryngospasm and subsequent acute airway obstruction.

8.3 Croup

Laryngotracheobronchitis ('croup') is a viral infection that affects children. Whilst often mild with no long-term sequelae, it **may present as life-threatening airway compromise**.

Pathophysiology

The most common causal organism is **parainfluenza virus (~80%)**, which is usually transmitted by respiratory droplets or through contamination of hands.

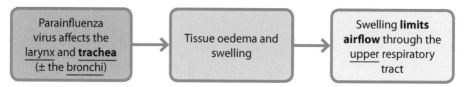

Parainfluenza virus affects the larynx and **trachea** (± the bronchi) → Tissue oedema and swelling → Swelling **limits airflow** through the upper respiratory tract

Epidemiology and risk factors

- Affects children **between the ages of 6 months and 3 years**
- **Most prevalent in late autumn**
- There is a slight **male preponderance** of 1.4:1

Diagnosis and investigation

Hx
- There is often an **antecedent history of viral URTI** symptoms, which progress over days into a characteristic **'barking' cough**.
- The child will often have a **hoarse cry** and an **inspiratory stridor**.
- In severe cases, symptoms of respiratory distress are present.
- In all cases, these **symptoms are worse, or only present, when the child is distressed**.

Ex
- **Fever.**
- **Look** for respiratory distress (*Fig. 8.5*) (↑RR, nasal flaring, tracheal tug, intercostal recession ± cyanosis).
- Listen for **inspiratory stridor**.
- ↓ air entry in severe cases.

DDx
Bacterial tracheitis is an uncommon condition caused by *S. aureus*, which presents with 'croup-like' features with ↑↑ purulent secretions.

Laryngoscopy is diagnostic. Emergency management of the airway and antibiotics are required.

Ix
In general, croup is a **clinical diagnosis** so investigations are not routinely ordered.

Management

Admit if <6 months old, graded 'severe', stridor at rest, respiratory distress or the child looks very unwell. In these patients, the following treatment is advised:

- Give **oxygen** to maintain saturations between 94 and 98%.
- A single **dose of corticosteroid**.
- **Nebulized adrenaline 1:1000** 0.4ml/kg (up to 5ml). Effects last for ~2 hours.

OSCE tips 2: Westley scoring system

This can be used to grade severity of croup. It is based on the clinical features including:

(i) inspiratory stridor

(ii) intercostal muscle recession

(iii) reduced air entry

(iv) presence of cyanosis and

(v) altered consciousness.

8.4 Bronchiolitis

Bronchiolitis is a **common** viral **lower respiratory** tract **infection** of **infants** between **2 and 6 months** of age and is the **leading cause of hospital admission in children**.

Pathophysiology

Infection of lower respiratory tract →

- Cell necrosis
- Inflammation
- Oedema
- ↑ Mucus secretion

→

- Hyperinflation
- ↑ Airway resistance
- Atelectasis
- Ventilation:perfusion mismatch

Epidemiology and risk factors

- **75% caused** by **respiratory syncytial virus (RSV)**; others include human metapneumovirus, adenovirus and parainfluenza virus.
- **Peak** incidence in **winter months** (November to March).
- **2–3**% infants **admitted** to hospital each year due to bronchiolitis.

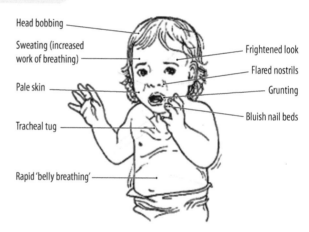

Head bobbing
Sweating (increased work of breathing)
Pale skin
Tracheal tug
Rapid 'belly breathing'
Frightened look
Flared nostrils
Grunting
Bluish nail beds

Fig. 8.5: Signs of respiratory distress.

Table 8.4: Risk factors for severe disease of bronchiolitis
Prematurity (born <37 weeks' gestation)
Chronic lung disease of prematurity
Immunodeficiency
Congenital/acquired lung disease (e.g. cystic fibrosis)
Congenital cardiac disease

Diagnosis and investigations

- **Symptoms** typically **peak** at **2–3 days** and **resolve** within **1–2 weeks**.

Hx
- Usually begin with coryzal **symptoms** of a **viral URTI** (**fever, rhinorrhoea** and **cough**).
- Followed by lower respiratory tract symptoms: **paroxysmal dry cough and dyspnoea** ± **wheeze**.
- May present with **vomiting** + **not taking feeds**.
- Ask about **apnoeic episodes** as this is a sign of severe disease.

Ex
- *Baseline observations*:
  - Fever, ↑HR, ↑RR ± ↓SpO$_2$
- *General observation*
  - **look for signs of respiratory distress** (see *Fig. 8.5*) + **dehydration**
- **Respiratory examination**
  - widespread **fine inspiratory crackles**
  - widespread **wheeze**
  - **hyperinflation** (palpable liver/spleen)

Ix
- In all cases, a **nasopharyngeal aspirate (NPA) is taken for rapid RSV testing** (useful mainly for **seclusion** on **wards** to prevent spread and **research** purposes).
- **In severe disease: bloods** and **CXR** (hyperinflation ± collapse).

DDx
- **Asthma**
- **Viral wheeze**
- **Pneumonia**

Management

Primary care	• A self-limiting illness usually conservatively managed at **home** with adequate **hydration** + **antipyrexial** medication (**paracetamol** or **ibuprofen**) – *most patients are in this category.*
Secondary care	• Consider **hospital admission** if: **poor feeding** (<50% usual intake), **signs** of **respiratory distress, sats ≤94%**, history of **apnoea, resp rate >70** breaths per minute.
	• **Mainstay** – supportive care including oxygen and nasogastric feeding where needed.
	• **Others** – bronchodilators, corticosteroids and antibiotics have **no significant benefit**.
	• nebulized hypertonic saline has shown good evidence to ↓hospital stay (*Cochrane: 2008 Oct 8;(4):CD006458*).
	• **nebulized adrenaline** may be beneficial.
	• **Vaccine** – palivizumab (monoclonal antibody) offered to high risk infants.

Pneumonia and lower respiratory tract infection

A lower respiratory tract infection (LRTI) is any infection below the level of the larynx and is a generalized term that, in practice, usually refers to bronchitis or pneumonia; it should be noted, however, that bronchiolitis and croup are also LRTIs. By definition, the presence of symptoms and signs of pneumonia **without** radiological changes is termed an LRTI, whilst the **presence** of radiological changes is termed pneumonia.

Pathophysiology

- An **inflammatory cascade** is triggered, leading to **increased vascular permeability**, with:
  - subsequent loss of plasma into the alveoli, leading to **reduced airspace and consolidation**
  - **airway narrowing** due to tissue oedema and increased production of mucus.

Table 8.5: Aetiological organisms in pneumonia/LRTI

Bacterial – typical	• *S. pneumoniae, H. influenzae, S. aureus, K. pneumoniae*
Bacterial – atypical	• *M. pneumoniae, L. pneumophila, C. pneumoniae*
Viral	• Influenza A, RSV, VZV, hMPV

Epidemiology and risk factors

- LRTIs have an estimated incidence of **~30 per 1000 children per year**.

Table 8.6: Risk factors for LRTI/pneumonia

Exposure to infected children	• As transmission is by direct inoculation or respiratory aerosol
Preterm birth	• Due to underdevelopment of the lungs
Cigarette smoke	• A significant risk factor for respiratory illness in children

Clinical features

Symptoms

- **In neonates, localizing symptoms to the chest are rare**; consequently, LRTI should **always** be considered in an unwell, febrile child.
- Symptoms of an **URTI commonly precede the illness** (see *Section 8.1*).
- The child will be **febrile** and have other **non-specific symptoms**.
- **Cough is the most common** symptom. Although classically productive of **purulent sputum**, this is *commonly absent in younger children*.

Signs

- Baseline observations will reveal **fever ± tachypnoea ± reduced SpO$_2$**.
- The patients **look unwell**. Look for signs of respiratory distress (see *Fig. 8.5*).
- Palpation and percussion: often omitted on very young children but, if done, signs may mimic those of adult disease (**reduced chest expansion** and **dull** percussion note).
- Auscultation: listen for **coarse crackles**, **asymmetry of air entry**, **bronchial breath sounds** or **focal wheeze**.

Investigation and diagnosis

Hx
- A febrile child with a cough ± preceding URTI symptoms.

Ex
- An unwell child with signs of respiratory distress.
- Chest auscultation may reveal localizing signs of infection.

Ix
- Investigations are mainly required to **identify the causal organism and therefore allow targeted therapy.**
- A **sputum culture** may be taken, although this is rarely positive.
- Bloods: **raised WCC** indicates infection and a blood **culture** may be useful.
- A **CXR may show consolidation** (*Fig. 8.6*), but does not reliably differentiate between viral and bacterial causes.

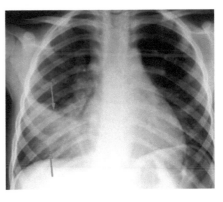

Fig. 8.6: Right middle lobe pneumonia in a 2-year-old.

DDx
- Asthma
- Bronchiolitis
- Inhaled foreign body
- Cardiac disease
- Gastro-oesophageal reflux disease (GORD)

Management

- *Most of these patients can be managed at home with close observation*; however, admit children who **look very unwell** or have significant **co-morbidity**.
- Simple **analgesics and anti-pyretics** (paracetamol and/or ibuprofen) are of benefit.
- Definitive treatment is with **antibiotics**.
  - for mild disease, which accounts for the vast majority of cases, PO amoxicillin is typically given for 3 days
  - admit children with sats <92%, RR >70, ↑↑HR, ↑CRT or apnoea/grunting.

Clinical pharmacology – Reye syndrome

Although paracetamol and ibuprofen are commonly used analgesics in children, there is concern about using aspirin, due to its association with Reye syndrome: an acute, non-inflammatory encephalopathy and fatty degeneration of the liver.

ASPIRIN SHOULD NOT BE USED FOR THOSE UNDER 16 YEARS OF AGE IN THE UK

8.6 Aspirated foreign body

Aspiration of larger foreign bodies (FB) will present with acute airway obstruction. Here, we discuss aspiration of smaller FB that move distal to the carina.

Pathophysiology

- Typically the causal FB is a **food item**, although older children tend to aspirate non-food items, such as paper clips and coins.
- Distal to the carina, the right and left main bronchi are symmetrical <15 y/o, so FB may be found either side.

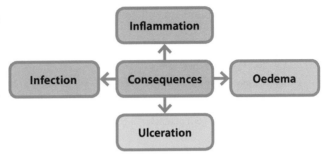

Fig. 8.7: Consequences of FB aspiration.

Epidemiology and risk factors

- 80% of cases are in **those under 3 years**.
- **Neurological disorders** increase the likelihood of aspiration.

Diagnosis

Hx
- A sudden episode of **coughing ± choking ± crying.**
- **Unwitnessed (~10–20%)** and a high index of suspicion is therefore required → delayed diagnosis may be fatal.
- The most common symptoms are **cough, wheeze and dyspnoea ± those of secondary infection.**

Ex
- Baseline observations: **fever, tachycardia, tachypnoea** ± low SaO_2.
- **Look for signs of respiratory distress** (nasal flaring, tracheal tug, intercostal recession and abdominal breathing ± cyanosis).
- Auscultation → **widespread fine inspiratory crackles.**

Ix
A **CXR**:
- **Radio-opaque** in ~10–20% of cases.
- **If radiolucent**, sequelae of the obstruction are seen → **atelectasis, unilateral hyperinflation** (air cannot leave the affected lung) or secondary **pneumonia**.

Bronchoscopy is gold standard for diagnosis (most FBs **not** seen on CXR).

Management

- Bronchoscopy for retrieval of the FB.
- If choking, manage as per the paediatric basic life support course instructions.
- **Prevention**:
  - avoidance of easily aspirated foods until the child is able to chew safely
  - feed sitting upright
  - avoid play whilst eating
  - keep small objects out of reach.

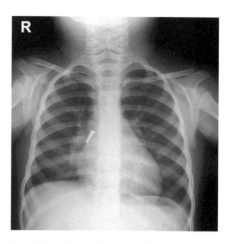

Fig. 8.8: CXR showing a screw in right main bronchus.

Paediatric choking algorithm

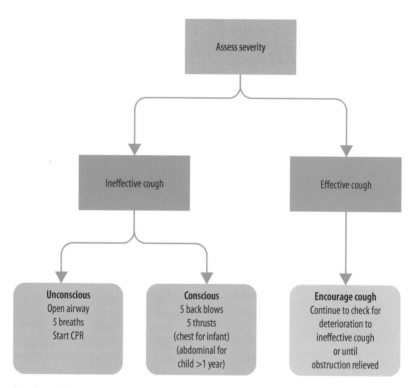

Reproduced with the kind permission of the Resuscitation Council (UK).

Pertussis (whooping cough)

Pertussis ('whooping cough' or '100 day cough') is a **notifiable** disease. Despite high uptake of the vaccine, pertussis is not uncommon, with 4341 confirmed cases in England in 2017.

Pathophysiology

- Spread via **respiratory droplets**, *Bordetella pertussis* is a **highly** contagious organism.
- Infection **spreads to bronchi and bronchioles** where an exudate forms. This **exudate can compromise the small airways**, predisposing to atelectasis and pneumonia.

Epidemiology and risk factors

Age less than 6 months	• Due to incomplete immunity
Contact with infected children	• Due to respiratory droplet spread

Diagnosis

Hx			
Catarrhal		**Symptoms closely** mimic those of an URTI.
Paroxysmal	TIME ↓ ↓ ↓ ↓	The cough is **dry, hacking and prolonged**, with the child **continuously** coughing until they have **completely emptied their lungs**. This is then **followed by an inspiratory 'whoop'**, which is produced by the child forcefully inspiring. Note, the child will typically **turn red in the face** and flail their limbs during episodes.
Convalescent		The child will be left with **a persistent** cough, **lasting up to 3 months ('100 days')**.

Ex
- The child **looks unwell**.
- Intense coughing may cause **petechiae on the face** (*Fig. 8.9*).
- Children are commonly **afebrile**.

Ix
- A **pernasal swab** is taken for diagnosis.
- ↑WCC with **high lymphocytes**.
- CXR may show perihilar infiltrates ± atelectasis.

OSCE tips 3: Petechiae on face

Intense bouts of coughing or crying can cause a petechial rash in the distribution of the SVC; therefore, petechiae confined to this area are unlikely to represent meningococcal disease.

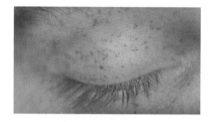

Fig. 8.9: Petechiae indicative of pertussis.

Management

- Treatment is **supportive**, ensuring good hydration, nutrition and oxygenation.
- **Antibiotics do not alter the clinical course** and are therefore rarely indicated.

Asthma

Affecting 15–20% of children, asthma is the most common chronic condition in children and is consequently seen very often as a student, in clinics, A&E and on the wards. The clinical picture seen is similar to that of adult disease; however, management is different and paediatric guidelines should be used.

Pathophysiology

- Asthma is a **chronic inflammatory condition** affecting the airways, characterized **by paroxysmal, reversible airway narrowing** and **airway hyper-responsiveness**.
- Pathological changes occur as shown in *Fig. 8.10*.
- This process may be initiated by a large number of **allergens** – classically cold air, exercise, viral illness, pollen, animal dander, dust mites and cigarette smoke – but it may also be non-specific.

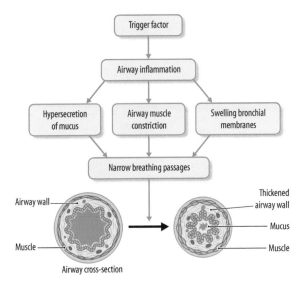

Fig. 8.10: Asthma pathophysiology.

Epidemiology and risk factors

- Peaks **between 5 and 15 years** of age. *Before 5 years, definitive diagnosis is difficult and therefore often intentionally delayed.*

Table 8.7: Major risk factors for asthma	
History of atopy	• Conditions such as eczema, allergic rhinitis and food allergy
Family history	• In a first-degree relative

Clinical features

Symptoms

- Expiratory **wheezing, often with a trigger**.
- Non-productive **cough**, classically **worse at night**.
- **Dyspnoea** and **chest tightness**, particularly on exertion.
- Features of **atopy** (allergic rhinitis, eczema, food allergy).
- Symptoms are often **recurrent**.

Signs – chronic

- On inspection, look for **eczematous skin changes** (particularly in the flexures), **hyperinflation** of the chest and, if a long history, **Harrison's sulcus** – a permanent horizontal groove inferior to the costal margin.
- Patients are often well between attacks and the remainder of the examination is therefore usually unremarkable.

Signs – acute

- **Severity** should be determined promptly using parameters in *Table 8.8*.
- Look for signs of **respiratory distress** and inspect for chest **hyperinflation**.
- Palpate for **reduced chest expansion**.
- Air entry will be equal but there will be **widespread polyphonic wheeze** across the chest. *A quiet or silent chest is indicative of life-threatening disease*.

OSCE tips 4: Asthma vs. viral-induced wheeze	
Asthma	**Viral wheeze**
Precipitated by 'triggers'	Precipitated by viral infection
May be wheezy between bouts	Symptom-free between bouts
Symptoms persistent >5 y/o	Symptoms most common <3 y/o
Responds to β_2-agonist predictably	Unpredictable response
History of atopy and FH of asthma or atopy	

Investigation and diagnosis

Table 8.8: Determining the severity of an acute asthma exacerbation	
Acute severe	**Life-threatening –** only ONE required
<ul><li>Peak expiratory flow rate (PEFR) 33–50% with SpO$_2$ <92%</li><li>Inability to complete sentences in single breath</li><li>HR >125 (>5 y/o) or >140 (2–5 y/o).</li><li>RR >30 (>5 y/o) or >40 (2–5 y/o).</li></ul>	<ul><li>PEFR <33% with SpO$_2$ <92%</li><li>Hypotension</li><li>Cyanosis</li><li>Silent chest or poor respiratory effort</li><li>Exhaustion</li><li>Confusion</li><li>Coma</li></ul>

Hx
- A wheezy child, over the age of 5, with chest tightness, nocturnal cough and the absence of concurrent URTI symptoms (viral-induced wheeze).
- Enquire about trigger factors.
- A personal or family history of asthma or atopy should be sought.

Ex
- Acutely, the child is in obvious respiratory distress and has widespread polyphonic wheeze.
- The severity of the exacerbation should be accurately assessed.
- The presence of **one** life-threatening symptom should be carefully looked for.
- Chronically, children may demonstrate signs of atopy and, in severely affected children, may develop chest hyperinflation and Harrison's sulcus.

Ix
- Diagnosis is often clinical in children.
- **Decide if there is a high, intermediate or low probability** of asthma:
  - **Low/intermediate:** if child able to tolerate **spirometry (typically ≥5 y/o)**, consider testing the lung function (for reversibility with a bronchodilator) and for **atopy** (RAST testing).
  - **High** or not tolerant of testing: trial of treatment.

DDx
- Viral-induced wheeze (see *OSCE tips 4*)
- Allergic rhinitis
- Bronchiolitis
- Gastro-oesophageal reflux
- If from birth, consider CF or congenital heart disease

Management

- Chronic management is based on the BTS/SIGN Stepwise Approach. Treatment is 'stepped up' if poorly controlled.

Table 8.9: Stepwise management of asthma in children, based on BTS/SIGN guidelines

	Step 1	Step 2	Step 3	Step 4	Step 5
<5 years	Inhaled short-acting β_2-agonist	Add inhaled steroid 200–400 mcg/day	± leukotriene receptor antagonist (montelukast)	Refer to paediatrician for specialist management	
5–12 years	Inhaled short-acting β_2-agonist	Add inhaled steroid 200–400 mcg/day	Add inhaled long-acting β_2-agonist ± montelukast or theophylline	Increase inhaled steroid to 800mcg/day	Commence oral steroid and refer to paediatrician

Oxygen

- **High-flow oxygen** in those with severe exacerbations or saturations <94%, aiming for a target of 94–98%

Bronchodilators

- **Inhaled β_2-agonists** delivered via a metered dose inhaler + spacer are first line; however, a nebulizer may be used
- If symptoms don't improve, add **ipratropium bromide** (250mcg)
- In children with a short duration of symptoms, who have sats <92%, consider adding 150mg **magnesium sulphate**

Steroids

- **Give steroids early**. Use 20mg prednisolone in children aged 2–5 and 30–40mg in those >5 years

Second line

- In children who have not responded initially to inhaled β_2-agonists, consider a **single IV bolus of salbutamol** (15mcg/kg over 10 minutes)
- Aminophylline is rarely indicated, and should be used only when severe/life-threatening asthma is unresponsive to maximal doses of bronchodilators and steroids

Fig. 8.11: Management of acute exacerbations of asthma. As per BTS guidelines (2014) for children >2 y/o.

Cystic fibrosis

Cystic fibrosis (CF) is a common, genetic, life-limiting condition and most patients will die in their 30s and 40s.

Pathophysiology

- An autosomal recessive genetic mutation in the *CFTR* gene on chromosome 7, which produces the CFTR protein.
- Its ordinary function is two-fold:
  1. To promote movement of chloride (Cl^-) ions down their concentration gradient:
     - They are found at the apical membranes of epithelial cell (in the lungs, pancreatic ducts, gastrointestinal tract, biliary tree and vas deferens) and so, in most instances, the Cl^- gradient drives Cl^- **out of cells and into the secretions**.
     - In sweat glands, which produce sweat with a high concentration of Cl^- (not CFTR protein-dependent), the role of CFTR is to **re-absorb Cl^- into** the cells. This re-absorption is impaired in patients with CF.
  2. To inhibit the effect of the epithelial sodium channel, an ion transporter which moves Na^+ (and subsequently water, which follows it) from the secretions and into the cells. When there is a mutation in the CFTR protein this inhibitory effect is lost and, therefore, Na^+ moves intracellularly.
- These changes lead to reduced Cl^-, Na^+ and H_2O in the secretions (with the exception of sweat, which has higher Cl^-), which are therefore **thicker and more viscous**.
- This affects the following systems:

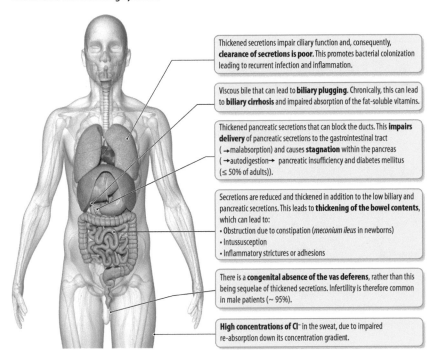

Thickened secretions impair ciliary function and, consequently, **clearance of secretions is poor.** This promotes bacterial colonization leading to recurrent infection and inflammation.

Viscous bile that can lead to **biliary plugging.** Chronically, this can lead to **biliary cirrhosis** and impaired absorption of the fat-soluble vitamins.

Thickened pancreatic secretions that can block the ducts. This **impairs delivery** of pancreatic secretions to the gastrointestinal tract (→malabsorption) and causes **stagnation** within the pancreas (→autodigestion→ pancreatic insufficiency and diabetes mellitus (≤ 50% of adults)).

Secretions are reduced and thickened in addition to the low biliary and pancreatic secretions. This leads to **thickening of the bowel contents,** which can lead to:
- Obstruction due to constipation (*meconium ileus* in newborns)
- Intussusception
- Inflammatory strictures or adhesions

There is a **congenital absence of the vas deferens**, rather than this being sequelae of thickened secretions. Infertility is therefore common in male patients (~ 95%).

High concentrations of Cl^- in the sweat, due to impaired re-absorption down its concentration gradient.

Fig. 8.12: Body systems affected by CF.

Epidemiology and risk factors

- Most prevalent in Caucasians, with an incidence of 1:2500 and a carrier rate of 1:25, but recognized in other ethnic groups also.
- Family history is the only significant risk factor.

Clinical features

- Clinical features of CF vary depending on age, but most will be related to sinopulmonary or gastrointestinal disease. The most common features for each age group are indicated as follows: infants (*), early childhood (†) and late childhood/adolescence (‡) in *Table 8.10*.

Table 8.10: Clinical features of cystic fibrosis		
System	**Symptoms**	**Signs**
Pulmonary	• Recurrent respiratory **infections***†‡ (initially *S. aureus* and *H. influenzae*; later, *P. aeruginosa*) • Chronic **cough***†‡ • Chronic sputum production • **Wheeziness***†‡ • Bronchiectasis†	• **Nasal polyps** in childhood are highly suggestive of CF† • Finger **clubbing** • **Crepitations** in the chest*†‡ • **Upper lobe wheeze** • Chest **hyperinflation**
Gastrointestinal	• **Meconium ileus*** (≤20% of newborns with CF) • **Failure to thrive*** • Rectal prolapse† • Features of obstruction	• Protuberant abdomen
Pancreatic	• Malabsorption* • **Steatorrhoea*** • Pancreatitis (recurrent) • Diabetes mellitus‡	• **Failure to thrive***
Biliary	• Prolonged neonatal jaundice* • **Malabsorption*** • Features of chronic liver disease‡	• **Failure to thrive*** • Features of liver disease: jaundice, portal hypertension or oesophageal varices‡
Urogenital	• **Infertility** due to congenital bilateral absence of the vas deferens (CBAVD)‡	• Infertile but normal sexual function otherwise • Undescended testicle • Hydrocele

Investigation and diagnosis

Ix

- The essential investigation is a **chloride sweat test**. In patients with CF, because the Cl⁻ ions are not reabsorbed from the sweat, it has a higher than normal Cl⁻ concentration. A **level of >60mmol/L** confirms the diagnosis.
- This can be **confirmed with genetic testing** for the *CFTR* gene.
- Bloods are usually taken and, alongside the routine tests, you may wish to look for the following:
  - fasting glucose or HbA1C – ?diabetes mellitus
  - vitamin A, D and E levels – ?malabsorption of the fat-soluble vitamins
- **CXR.**
- Pulmonary function testing – the **FEV₁** is a useful measure and is checked on a regular basis and *declines with disease progression*.

Management

- The management of these children is complex and requires **tertiary referral** and involvement of the **multidisciplinary team**, with the overall aims being to slow lung disease progression and ensure adequate nutrition.
- Respiratory disease:
  - **chest physiotherapy** twice daily
  - prophylactic **antibiotics** with additional doses available for infective exacerbations
  - **mucolytics** can be used to thin secretions, making them easier to expectorate:
    - dornase alfa – a recombinant DNAse that cleaves neutrophilic DNA in the sputum
    - hypertonic saline – osmotically draws fluid into the airway mucus
  - there is some benefit gained from the use of **bronchodilators**
  - monitor the **FEV₁ regularly** in children old enough to perform this
  - in end-stage disease, the only therapeutic option is **lung transplantation**.
- Gastrointestinal disease:
  - **high-calorie intake** (~130% of recommended daily intake).
- Pancreatic disease:
  - pancreatic enzymes (**Creon**)
  - screen for diabetes mellitus regularly and, if diagnosed, treatment is usually with subcutaneous insulin.
- Biliary disease:
  - fat-soluble **vitamin supplements** (A, D and E)
  - if biliary cirrhosis ensues, **liver transplantation** is an option in those with good pulmonary function.
- Fertility:
  - *in vitro* **fertilization** is an option for sterile males, using extraction techniques to retrieve viable sperm from the patient's testes.
  - genetic counselling is important, as children of affected patients will be carriers of the *CFTR* gene (or potentially affected if the patient's partner also has the gene).

Chapter 9

Gastrointestinal disorders

Feeding, overfeeding and weaning

This is an important topic often overlooked by medical students, but a good understanding of a baby's diet can help clinically in identifying the common presentation of vomiting due to overfeeding, as well as in giving new parents advice.

Table 9.1: Feeding and weaning schedule	
0–6 months	• **Milk:** babies are fed entirely on milk, ideally from the breast although formula milk is also acceptable. They need nothing else for the first 6 months. • **Cow's milk:** should not be given at all as it can cause *iron-deficiency anaemia*. • **Water:** all water must be boiled and left to cool first. Typically, babies will not need water as all of their fluid comes from milk (although it is needed to make formula).
6 months	• **Milk:** continue with breast or formula milk. • **Cow's milk:** may be mixed with food, but not given as a drink. • **Water:** no longer needs to be boiled first and, as solids are introduced, may be given if the child is thirsty. Introduce cups for drinking. • **Solids:** begin to introduce solids ('**weaning**'), initially mashed or soft-cooked. As the child becomes more confident and better able to coordinate chewing and swallowing, firmer foods can be introduced.
~9 months	• **Milk:** continue with breast or formula milk, but at a reduced amount and with reduced time on the breast/bottle. • **Cow's milk:** may be mixed with food, but not given as a drink. • **Water:** no longer needs to be boiled first and should be given if the child is thirsty. • **Solids:** the child should be heading towards 3 meals per day.
12 months	• **Milk:** continue with breast milk if desired, but formula should be stopped in favour of cow's milk. • **Cow's milk:** may be taken as a drink, but should be full fat and from a cup. • **Water:** from the tap and drunk from a cup. • **Solids:** 3 meals per day.

Overfeeding – a diagnosis of exclusion

Overfeeding should be considered in children who are fed **≥200ml/kg/day (normal = 150ml/kg/day)**. Children typically present with posseting or vomiting, *without any other symptoms*. On examination, the child is well, gaining weight normally, well hydrated and has no findings on examination. Treatment is with education.

Gastroenteritis

Gastroenteritis is very common in children and a significant cause of morbidity in developed countries. In the developing world, it accounts for ~20% of childhood deaths under 5 years old, thus illustrating the importance of good management of these patients.

Pathophysiology

- Viral causes account for ~60% of cases and are responsible for winter epidemics, with rotavirus (55%) and norovirus the main agents.
  - Bacterial causes include: *Campylobacter* spp., *salmonella* spp., *shigella* spp. and *E. coli* O157:H7.

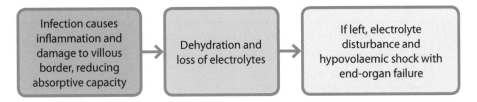

Epidemiology and risk factors

Clinical features

Symptoms

- Usually begins with non-specific symptoms such as low grade fever, followed by vomiting and/or diarrhoea.
  - Viral is typically non-bloody, but haematochezia may occur with *Shigella*, *Campylobacter* or *E. coli* O157:H7.
- Child may complain of abdominal pain.
- Of note, febrile convulsions may occur with *Shigella* infection.

Table 9.2: Risk factors for gastroenteritis
Age under 5 years
Poor hygiene
Poverty
Contact with infected children
Daycare attendance
Winter months
Lack of breastfeeding

Signs

- Baseline observations may reveal a fever.
- Formally assess the child's hydration status and check their height, weight and head circumference.
- The abdomen is usually soft and non-distended, but may be tender (no rebound or guarding).
- On auscultation, the bowel sounds are often hyperactive.
- Undo the nappy and check any stool and the anus for redness.

OSCE tips 1: *E. coli* O157:H7 and haemolytic uraemic syndrome

Due to its production of Shiga-toxin, ~10% of children with *E. coli* O157:H7 infection will go on to develop haemolytic uraemic syndrome (HUS); a condition characterized by the presence of acute kidney injury, haemolysis and thrombocytopenia.

Investigation and diagnosis

Hx
- Diarrhoea and vomiting with a low grade fever.
- Diarrhoea *may* be bloody.

Ex
- It is essential to check the hydration status of these children.
- The abdomen may be tender but there is no peritonism present.
- Bowel sounds are hyperactive.

Ix
- Generally, a clinical diagnosis.
- If the stool is bloody, or if profound dehydration is noted, consider:
  - stool MC&S.
  - bloods: FBC (raised WCC) and U&E (identify metabolic derangement).

DDx
- Inflammatory bowel disease (IBD)
- Lactose intolerance
- Intussusception
- Appendicitis
- Mesenteric adenitis
- UTI
- Pyelonephritis

Management

- Encourage the mother to continue breastfeeding/formula feeding as normal, and push oral fluids (if >6 months). Antibiotics and anti-diarrhoeals are **not** routinely prescribed.
- Add an anti-emetic if vomiting is prominent (typically ondansetron).
- Fluid management is dependent on hydration status (see *Table 9.3*).

Table 9.3: Fluid management required in gastroenteritis based on % dehydration

Clinically hydrated	Offer oral rehydration salts (ORS) as maintenance
<5%	Give 50ml/kg ORS PO over 4 hours to rehydrate, then offer maintenance as above
5–10%	Give 100ml/kg ORS PO over 4 hours to rehydrate, then offer maintenance as above • Use NG tube if not tolerated
>10%	Rehydrate with 20ml/kg IV normal 0.9% saline over 1 hour and then offer maintenance as above

OSCE tips 2: Advice for parents (NICE 2009, CG84)

- Provide a 'safety net' – advise parents how to spot Red Flag symptoms for dehydration and shock.
- Children can usually be safely managed at home and symptoms tend to improve within 5–7 days.
- Encourage plenty of fluids (ORS if required) and avoid fruit and carbonated drinks.
- Reintroduce the child's normal diet as soon as they can tolerate it.
- Contact a healthcare professional if dehydration or symptoms not resolving.

Gastro-oesophageal reflux (GOR) has a prevalence of 2–10% in babies and usually presents before the age of 4 months.

Pathophysiology

- Causes are multifactorial, as shown in *Fig. 9.1*.
- Post-prandially, there is effortless regurgitation of gastric contents into the oesophagus and mouth.
- This can lead to irritation of the oesophagus or respiratory complications, such as cough or wheeze.

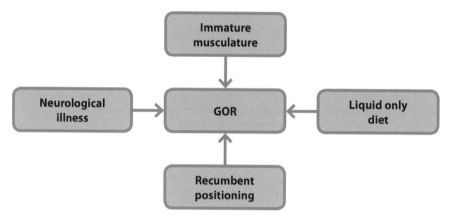

Fig. 9.1: Overall causes of GOR in children.

Epidemiology and risk factors

Table 9.4: Risk factors for gastro-oesophageal reflux	
Obesity	• One of the most significant risk factors
Increased intra-gastric pressure	• Such as pyloric stenosis and other causes of outflow obstruction
Neurodevelopmental abnormalities	• Such as cerebral palsy and Down syndrome
Oesophageal abnormalities	• Such as hiatal herniae

Clinical features

Symptoms
- Regurgitation or 'effortless' vomiting, typically occurring *post-prandially*.
- Abdominal pain *post-prandially*: if left, this may manifest as feeding difficulties and failure to thrive (FTT).
- If complications are present, oesophagitis may present as haematemesis or dysphagia.
- Enquire about torticollis or opisthotonus (hyperextension of the back and neck, forming a 'reverse bow'; *Fig. 3.14*). This is seen in Sandifer syndrome, which occurs in ~1% of patients with GOR, in which these tonic symptoms commonly follow feeding.

Signs
- Check the infant's height, weight and head circumference to identify FTT (see *Section 4.1*).
- Other examination findings are usually essentially normal.

Investigation and diagnosis

Hx
- Regurgitation/vomiting, classically post-prandially.
- There may be pain at the same time, which, in these infants, tends to manifest as crying.
- Enquire about torticollis and opisthotonus.

Ex
- Ensure the child is growing adequately.

Ix
- Usually a clinical diagnosis, based on the child's age (≤4/12), the history and its relationship with feeding.
- If unclear, a 24-hour oesophageal pH study, barium meal (to look for anatomical abnormalities) or endoscopy may be indicated.

DDx
- Overfeeding
- Gastritis, gastroenteritis
- Food allergy such as cow's milk protein
- Hiatal herniae
- Pyloric stenosis
- Malrotation
- Meningitis
- UTI

Management

Non-pharmacological	Reassure parents that *this is a common condition that tends to resolve with age*. Initially, parents should **avoid overfeeding**, try **reducing the volume** of feeds but increasing their frequency, encourage **upright positioning**, and **properly wind** the infant (See *OSCE tips 3*).
Pharmacological	• Feed thickeners can be trialled but evidence is poor. • Gaviscon Infant is usually given initially. • Omeprazole: PPIs are generally *last-line* management, as there is an increased risk of community-acquired pneumonia, gastroenteritis and necrotizing enterocolitis. • Ranitidine: H2RAs may be beneficial.
Surgical	• Nissen's fundoplication is reserved for those with life-threatening complications of the disease.

OSCE tips 3: How to wind a baby

When young babies feed they often swallow air along with the milk, although this is more the case with bottle-fed babies. If left, this can cause discomfort and posseting. To wind a child, advise the parent to gently rub and/or pat on their child's back in one of the following positions:

1) on their chest with child's chin resting on parent's shoulder

2) sitting sideways on their lap, or

3) face down on their lap.

9.4 Infantile colic

This is a benign condition without any known underlying medical or surgical cause, presenting in between 10 and 30% of infants. It typically begins in the first few weeks of life and resolves spontaneously by 4–5 months of age.

Pathophysiology

- The pathophysiology of this condition is not clear.
- There is some evidence to suggest that these infants have higher motilin levels than usual, resulting in increased gastric and intestinal motility.

Epidemiology and risk factors

Table 9.5: Risk factors for infantile colic
Age under 5 months
Exposure to cigarette smoke
Formula-fed only

Rapid diagnosis – rule of 3s

Characterized by paroxysmal crying:
- that lasts >**3 hours** per episode
- on >**3 days** of the week
- for >**3 weeks**.

Diagnosis and investigations

Hx
- Paroxysms of crying, often worse in the afternoons and evenings.
- Flatus may be present and typically relieves the infant's symptoms.
- Other features as in *Fig. 9.2*.

Ex
- Infants are well and growing normally.
- There should be no other findings on examination.

Ix
- A clinical diagnosis.

DDx Any cause of excessive crying, which may include
- UTI
- Cow's milk protein intolerance
- GOR
- Anal fissure
- Intussusception
- Pyloric stenosis
- Acute otitis media
- Non-accidental injury (NAI)
- Meningitis

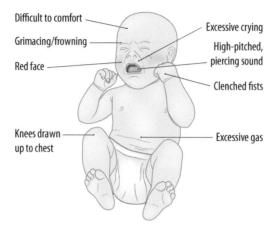

Difficult to comfort

Grimacing/frowning

Red face

Excessive crying

High-pitched, piercing sound

Clenched fists

Knees drawn up to chest

Excessive gas

Fig. 9.2: Clinical features of infantile colic.

Management

- Sadly, there is no definitive management for this condition, which can be very distressing for the child's parents: referral to peer support may therefore be helpful.
- It is advised that parents hold the baby throughout the crying episode.
- Bottle-fed infants may benefit from a hydrolysed formula, particularly if there is a suspicion that the diagnosis may be cow's milk protein intolerance.

Constipation

The cause of constipation in children is **functional** (that is, no organic causes are found) in ≤95% of cases; however, in a small number, an underlying condition is present. It is important therefore to *exclude any 'Red Flags'* for underlying neurological or surgical causes.

Pathophysiology and risk factors

Functional constipation will generally begin with a low-fibre, low-fluid diet resulting in hardening of the stool. A cycle, as illustrated in *Fig. 9.3*, may then begin.

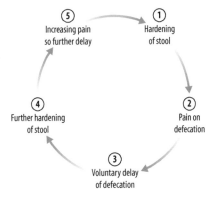

Fig. 9.3: The cycle that may follow an initial episode of hard stool in children.

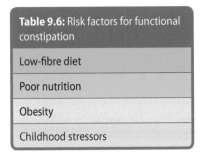

Table 9.6: Risk factors for functional constipation
Low-fibre diet
Poor nutrition
Obesity
Childhood stressors

Clinical features

Symptoms

- Painful passage of infrequent, hard stool.
- Overflow faecal incontinence is common and produces small volume, soft stool.
- Enquire about Red Flag Symptoms (see box) specifically.

Red Flag symptoms (NICE 2010, CG99)
Present from birth
Delayed passage of meconium (≥48 hours)
'Ribbon stools'
Neurological symptoms or signs, such as locomotor delay or falling over/abnormal gait in older children
Vomiting
Abdominal distension

Signs

- On inspection, the child is well, growing normally and has a normal gait.
- Palpation of the abdomen may reveal an indentable mass, usually in the left lower quadrant (LLQ).
- There is no gross distension.
- Examine for the below specifically:

Spine	Gluteal region	Perianal region	Lower limbs
Hairy patches or lipomata, indicative of spina bifida	Symmetry	No fissures and anatomically normal anus	Normal power, tone and reflexes

Investigation and diagnosis

Hx
- Infrequent, hard stool passed in the absence of any Red Flag symptoms.

Ex
- It is important to note that the child should be growing normally.
- There may be an indentable mass in the LLQ, but examination – which should include the back, perianal region and lower limbs – is otherwise normal.

Ix
- Usually a clinical diagnosis; however, if ongoing, consider:
  - blood tests for coeliac disease and hypothyroidism
  - plain abdominal X-ray or ultrasound
  - rectal biopsy (if Hirschsprung disease is suspected).

DDx
- In infants:
  - Hirschsprung disease
  - Cystic fibrosis
  - Hypothyroidism
  - Spinal dysraphism (i.e. spina bifida)
  - Anogenital anomalies such as imperforate anus (with a fistula)
- In older children:
  - Neuromuscular disorders (spinal muscular atrophy, cerebral palsy)
  - Hypothyroidism
  - Anorexia.

Management

- Pharmacological disimpaction is first line, if the child has significant faecal loading (overflow incontinence or indentable mass)
  - Polyethylene glycol 3350 (Movicol, an osmotic laxative) is used initially. Lactulose is an alternative.
  - If no improvement in 2 weeks, add a stimulant laxative such as senna.
- Maintenance: continue polyethylene glycol 3350. A stimulant may be added.
- All parents and children should receive dietary and lifestyle advice, to include:
  - regular, scheduled toileting
  - increasing dietary fibre and fluids
  - increasing exercise.

Clinical pharmacology: Commonly used laxatives in children		
Class	**Name**	**Mechanism of action**
Macrogols	Polyethylene glycol 3350 (Movicol)	Induces effect by retaining water in the stool. This softens the stool and increases its bulk, so increasing the frequency.
Osmotic	Lactulose	Broken down to lactic acid which raises the osmotic pressure of the bowel, so inducing its effect as described above.
Stimulant	Senna	Breakdown products are directly irritant to the bowel wall, causing increased fluid secretion and colonic motility.

Hirschsprung disease

Also known as aganglionic bowel, Hirschsprung disease is an important differential in neonates with delayed passage of meconium. Of these, ~50% with delayed passage have the disease.

Pathophysiology

- There is absence of ganglion cells in the bowel wall myenteric nerve plexus. *In utero*, these cells migrate in a craniocaudal fashion. Consequently, the distal bowel is affected most often (70% rectosigmoid, 20% rest of colon), with only 10% in the small bowel.
- Their absence results in a lack of effective peristalsis and muscle spasm, leading to impaired relaxation of the bowel wall and the internal anal sphincter.
- As a result, these children have a functional obstruction of their bowel.

Red Flag symptoms (NICE CG99 2010)

Due to stasis of faeces, there is *increased susceptibility to enterocolitis* (~12% of patients). If untreated, sepsis rapidly ensues and there is a mortality rate of 30–50%.

Epidemiology and risk factors

- ~1.6 per 100 000 live births, with a male preponderance of 2:1.
- The most significant association is with Down syndrome: up to 15% of those with Hirschsprung disease also have Down syndrome.

Clinical features

Symptoms

- Delayed passage of meconium (>48 hours) is the typical presentation.
- Vomiting, which will eventually become bilious.
- When stool is passed, it is usually foul (due to bacterial growth) and explosive.

Signs

- **If complicated by enterocolitis, the child will be febrile** – this is therefore an important sign.
- On inspection, the abdomen will be distended (see *Fig. 9.4.*)
- Palpation should be unremarkable – where tenderness is found, enterocolitis should be suspected.

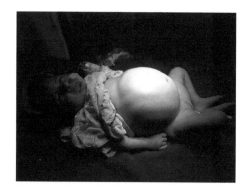

Fig. 9.4: Abdominal distension in a child with Hirschsprung disease.

Delayed passage of meconium

Meconium, the first stool a baby passes, is typically seen within 48 hours. The other important differential in these children is meconium ileus, of which 90% have cystic fibrosis.

Investigation and diagnosis

Hx
- Passage of meconium >48 hours ± vomiting.

Ex
- The abdomen is distended.
- At this point, you must ask yourself if it is complicated by necrotizing enterocolitis:
  - ?febrile ?abdominal tenderness

Ix
- Bloods: if the child is febrile. Raised WCC suggests possible enterocolitis.
- Plain abdominal X-ray (AXR): will show a picture of bowel obstruction, typically of the (distal) colon (see *Fig. 9.5*).
- Rectal biopsy: this is the definitive investigation. As the cells migrate distally, if a patient has Hirschsprung disease it will always be present in the rectum.

DDx
- Meconium ileus (?cystic fibrosis)

Management

- Acutely, stop enteral feeding (NBM) and so commence maintenance fluids IV.
  - Decompress the stomach and bowel by placing an NG tube and starting saline enemas.
  - If enterocolitis is present, start broad-spectrum antibiotics IV.
- Surgical resection of the aganglionic segment with a coloanal anastomosis is definitive (see *Fig. 9.6*).

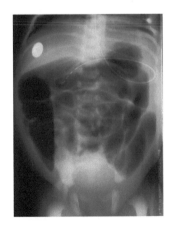

Fig. 9.5: AXR showing a picture of bowel obstruction. The aganglionic segment, however, is often of smaller diameter.

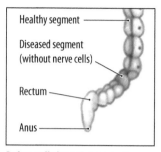

Healthy segment

Diseased segment
(without nerve cells)

Rectum

Anus

Before pull-through surgery: the
diseased segment doesn't push stool

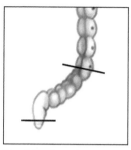

Step 1: the diseased segment
is removed

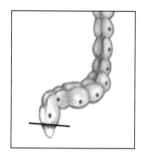

Step 2: the healthy segment is
attached to the remaining rectum

Fig. 9.6: The surgical procedure used for treating Hirschsprung disease.

Anal fissure

Epi Often <2 years old, but can occur at any age. A common cause of rectal bleeding in childhood.

Path Hard stool stretches the anal mucosa causing a tear, resulting in **pain during a bowel movement**. This has 2 consequences (i) **spasm** of the internal anal sphincter, causing ↓ blood flow and therefore poor healing, and (ii) **avoidance** of opening bowels → worsening constipation.

Hx Pain during defecation, which lasts minutes–hours. There are often small volumes of bright-red blood on the paper. Pain leads to toilet avoidance, thus worsening constipation and therefore pain.

Ex Fissures may be seen as a break in the anal mucosa, often in the posterior midline.

Ix Not required

Rx The aim of treatment is to **soften the stools**, so avoiding pain and sphincter spasm, and therefore allowing the fissure to heal. **Increasing fluid and fibre in the diet is required, as are laxatives** – all should be continued for ~1 month after symptoms resolve to permit complete healing. Additionally, sitting in a warm bath 2–3 times per day has been shown to increase healing. Surgery is occasionally required.

Threadworm (*Enterobius vermicularis*)

Epi A very common infection of childhood, typically affecting children from 5–10 years.

Path A **highly contagious** infection with the threadworm *Enterobius vermicularis*. These ~1cm worms live in the small bowel but migrate to the anus to lay eggs, which are **highly irritant and cause the child to scratch** the area. Eggs on their fingers can be passed to their mouth to re-infect them, or transferred elsewhere to infect others.

Hx Intense perianal itching, often worse at night. This disturbs sleep → behavioural problems. Small, thread-like worms **may** be seen in the perianal region.

Ex Excoriations ± worms present.

Ix If worms seen → not required. Otherwise, the **'tape-test'** is performed: the parent places a piece of sticky tape briefly on the child's anus first thing in the morning, which is then sent for microscopy.

Rx Definitive treatment is a dose of **antifungal**, typically mebendazole. Importantly, **measures should be taken to prevent transmission/re-infection for 2 weeks post-treatment, as the antifungal only kills live worms**. These include daily washing of bedding, fastidious hand hygiene, bathing every morning with cleansing of the perianal region and storing their toothbrushes out of reach.

9.8 Chronic diarrhoea

9.8.1 Cow's milk protein intolerance

Cow's milk protein intolerance (CMPI) is the most common childhood food allergy, affecting **2–7.5% of infants**. Happily, most children will grow out of the allergy in childhood.

Pathophysiology

- Cow's milk protein is found **predominantly in baby formula**, although there is speculation that small amounts of bovine milk protein can be found in maternal breast milk.
- CMPI is *either* a type I (immediate; IgE-mediated) or type IV (delayed; non-IgE-mediated) hypersensitivity reaction; **the former is most common**.
  - Up to 60% of affected infants will have a reaction **within 2 hours** of ingestion.
- The most significant risk factor for development of this condition is a **family history of parental or sibling atopy**, which increases the child's risk by 20–40%.

Clinical features

- The symptoms and signs vary depending on whether this is an IgE-mediated (immediate) or non-IgE-mediated (delayed) reaction to cow's milk.

Table 9.7: Features of cow's milk protein intolerance (modified from NICE CKS 2015)

	IgE-mediated	Non-IgE-mediated
Onset	Within 2 hours	Between 48 hours and 2 weeks
Dermatological	Pruritus and erythema	Pruritus and erythema
	Urticarial rash	*Eczematous* rash
	Angioedema (lips and face)	Angioedema unusual
Gastrointestinal	Nausea and vomiting	
	Colic	Colic, which may mimic infantile colic
	Diarrhoea	Chronic diarrhoea, which *may be bloody*
		Perianal redness
Respiratory	Lower respiratory symptoms, such as wheeze and dyspnoea	Lower respiratory symptoms, such as wheeze and dyspnoea
	Upper respiratory symptoms, such as sneezing, rhinorrhoea and nasal itching	

Investigation and diagnosis

Hx
- In those with IgE-mediated disease, symptoms of acute allergy within 2 hours of cow's milk ingestion.
- In children with non-IgE-mediated disease, features of atopy are more prominent.
- Ensure you ask about a family history of atopy.

Ex
- Is the child growing properly? Those with delayed type may fail to thrive.
- Perform a thorough examination of the skin for any rashes.
- Examine the gastrointestinal and respiratory systems.

Ix
- If IgE-mediated (immediate), **skin prick** or **specific IgE antibody blood ('RAST') testing** will confirm the diagnosis.
- If the non-IgE-mediated condition is suspected, eliminating cow's milk from the diet for 2–6 weeks is recommended.

DDx
- Other food allergy (such as lactose intolerance or food allergens – eggs, soya, wheat)
- Chronic gastrointestinal disease (IBD, GORD, coeliac disease, constipation with overflow)

Management

- Management is with **exclusion of cow's milk from the diet**, so these patients may benefit from a **dietetics referral**.
- First line is to switch the infant to a **hydrolysed formula**, although this is said to taste unpleasant so is not always well tolerated.
- If this is not tolerated, **soy milk can be given to infants >6 months old** (due to its weak oestrogenic effect), although there is some cross-reactivity.
- Over 5 years old, rice milk may be tried and in older children, oat milk, both of which should be fortified with calcium.
- Symptoms should resolve within ~1 week of treatment and, overall, CMPI will typically resolve within 1–2 years.

Skin prick and RAST testing

Skin prick testing is a safe, simple way to assess if a child has an IgE-mediated allergy to food or aero-allergens. A lancet is used to introduce a sample of the allergen into the skin; if the child is allergic, they will produce a wheal.

RAST (radioallergosorbent test) is a blood test that measures the serum levels of **allergen-specific** IgE, which go up in allergic individuals. It is beneficial in those where skin prick testing is difficult (i.e. infants), if skin prick testing is equivocal, or where there is a significant risk of causing anaphylaxis if skin prick testing is done.

9.8.2 Coeliac disease

Present in ~1% of the population, coeliac disease (CD) is an autoimmune disease triggered by gluten, a protein found in **wheat, barley and rye**.

Pathophysiology

- Gliadin, a glycoprotein extract from gluten, is the most important molecule in the pathophysiology of coeliac disease.
- In the bowel wall, gliadin is deamidated by tissue transglutaminase (tTG), which allows it to bind to HLA-DQ2 or DQ8 on antigen-presenting cells.
- This leads to activation of Th-cells. Th1-cells induce Tc-cells to cause damage to the bowel wall, resulting in the classical changes of **villous atrophy and crypt hyperplasia**. Th2-cells are responsible for inducing plasma cells to produce auto-antibodies anti-gliadin and anti-tTG.
- As a consequence, absorption of nutrients in the bowel is poor and, commonly, so is the **absorption of iron**.

Epidemiology and risk factors

Table 9.8: Risk factors for coeliac disease	
Family history of coeliac disease	• Increases risk of coeliac disease by ~10%
Type I diabetes mellitus	• Between 2 and 10% of patients with coeliac disease also have type 1 diabetes mellitus (T1DM)
IgA deficiency	• IgA deficiency is 10–15 times more common in these patients

Clinical features

Symptoms

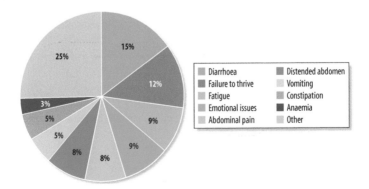

Fig. 9.7: The presenting symptom of children with coeliac disease (%).

Signs

- Check the child's growth.
- Children are often irritable.
- In older children, mouth ulcers and angular stomatitis are common (↓ iron).
- The child may be pale and there may be classical wasting of the buttocks with distension of the abdomen (see *Fig. 9.8*).

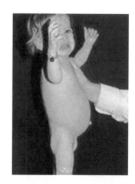

Investigation and diagnosis

Fig. 9.8: Abdominal distension with flattened, wasted buttocks.

Hx
- Chronic **diarrhoea**, which is often **offensive**, pale and may float in the pan.
- This may be associated with failure to thrive, abdominal bloating and pain.

Ex
- Assess the child's height, weight and head circumference.
- Look for abdominal bloating and wasting of the buttocks.
- In older children, look for dermatitis herpetiformis (see *OSCE tips 4*).

Ix
- Bloods:
  - FBC – there may be a **low Hb with low MCV** due to reduced iron absorption
  - auto-antibodies – **anti-tTG and anti-endomysial antibodies** (EMA)
  - HLA-DQ2/DQ8.
- Definitive diagnosis is with **jejunal biopsy**, which shows crypt hyperplasia and villous atrophy. This is done where blood tests are inconclusive or coeliac disease is suspected but the child is asymptomatic.

DDx
- IBD
- Irritable bowel syndrome (IBS)
- Autoimmune enteropathy
- Cystic fibrosis
- Bacterial overgrowth

Management

- Treatment is with a **gluten-free diet**, which excludes all wheat, barley and rye products; even small amounts are not permitted.
  - A dietitian referral is of value to this end.
- Supplementation of calcium and vitamin D may be required.

OSCE tips 4: Dermatitis herpetiformis

Dermatitis herpetiformis (DH) is an autoimmune dermatological condition that is strongly associated with CD: around 80% of patients with DH have histological changes consistent with CD, although only ~20% are symptomatic. It tends to present in middle age, but may also be present in children, so it is important to enquire about rashes when you see these patients.

The rash associated with DH (*Fig. 9.9*) has the following characteristics:

- Intensely pruritic
- Erythematous
- Papular
- Affects extensor surfaces (elbows/knees), scalp and buttocks.

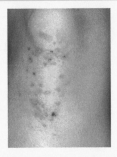

Fig. 9.9: Rash seen in DH.

9.8.3 Lactose intolerance

Lactose intolerance may be primary (lactase deficiency) or secondary; *the latter is more common in children*.

Pathophysiology

Pathophysiology of primary and secondary lactose intolerance		
	Primary	**Secondary**
1.	An autosomal recessive condition leading to reduction in lactase activity	Pathology of the GI tract – **typically viral gastroenteritis** – damages the villi of the small bowel and causes a reduction in the activity of lactase
2.	A reduction in lactase activity diminishes hydrolysis of lactose in the small bowel, so leaving it to pass into the colon unchanged	
3.	In the colon, it acts as an osmolyte, keeping water in the bowel; in addition, it is digested by bacteria to form short-chain fatty acids and gas	

Epidemiology and risk factors

- It is estimated that ~25% of Caucasians are lactose intolerant, rising significantly in other ethnic groups (≥75%).
- Symptoms of primary intolerance typically present after 6 years of age.

Table 9.9: Risk factors for lactose intolerance
Gastroenteritis (secondary)
Family history (primary)
Non-white ethnicity (primary)

Diagnosis and investigation

Hx
- **Watery** diarrhoea that follows gastroenteritis.
- Abdominal discomfort and ↑ flatus.

Ex
- Check the child is growing normally and is hydrated.
- Abdominal bloating or distension.

Ix
- Stool sample: for **pH (<6.0)** and reducing sugars.
- In older children, a hydrogen breath test or lactose tolerance test may be used.

DDx
- Cow's milk protein intolerance
- IBD
- IBS
- Gastroenteritis
- Coeliac disease
- Infantile colic
- Giardiasis
- Hyperthyroidism
- Meckel diverticulum

Management

- Switch to **lactose-free diet**/milk/formula.
  - This is not absolute and *varying degrees of lactose may be tolerated*
  - A **dietitian** referral will be required.
- Consider vitamin D and calcium supplementation.
- In secondary disease, **cow's milk can be reintroduced** once symptoms have resolved (weeks–months).

9.8.4 Toddler diarrhoea

Toddler diarrhoea is a very common cause of chronic diarrhoea in young children (between ~6 months and 5 years of age) who are otherwise well. It is self-limiting and without long-term significance.

Pathophysiology

The mechanisms underlying this condition are not well understood, but there is speculation that it is due to an exaggerated gastrocolic reflex.

Epidemiology and risk factors

The only risk factor for toddler diarrhoea is male sex.

Diagnosis and investigation

Hx
- Chronic diarrhoea, which **classically contains particles of undigested food** (often peas and carrots) ± mucus.
  - Stools tend to be firmer in the mornings.
- May be exacerbated by high-fibre diets and sugary (fruit) juices.

Ex
- The **examination is normal** and, importantly, the child's growth must be within normal limits.
- There must be no suggestion of malabsorptive disease present (such as weight loss, bloating or steatorrhoea).

Ix
- This is a clinical diagnosis of exclusion.

DDx
- Malabsorptive disease (IBD, coeliac, pancreatic insufficiency)
- Food allergy (cow's milk)
- Lactose intolerance

Management

- Reassurance is especially important, as parents are often understandably worried that their child has a serious illness. Highlight that this is also **not** a precursor to gastrointestinal illness as an adult and symptoms typically resolve by 4–5 years of age.
- There is no role for medication in the management of toddler diarrhoea.
- **Dietary amendments** may be of use:

Limit intake of:	Include:
Fruit juice; fizzy drinks	Full-fat milk
Grapes; raisins	All other fruit
Peas; baked beans; sweetcorn	All other vegetables
High-fibre cereals	Low fibre cereals
Low-fat dairy	Full-fat dairy

Adapted from Norfolk and Norwich University Hospitals NHS Foundation Trust.

Acute abdomen

Pyloric stenosis

Pathophysiology

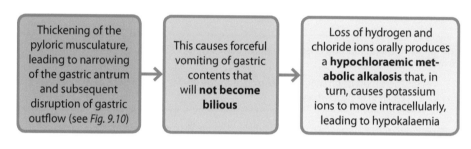

Thickening of the pyloric musculature, leading to narrowing of the gastric antrum and subsequent disruption of gastric outflow (see *Fig. 9.10*)	This causes forceful vomiting of gastric contents that will **not become bilious**	Loss of hydrogen and chloride ions orally produces a **hypochloraemic metabolic alkalosis** that, in turn, causes potassium ions to move intracellularly, leading to hypokalaemia

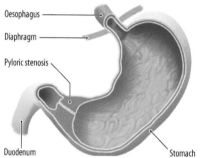

Oesophagus
Diaphragm
Pyloric stenosis
Duodenum
Stomach

Fig. 9.10: Pyloric stenosis.

Table 9.10: Risk factors for pyloric stenosis
Male sex
Family history

Epidemiology and risk factors

- Significantly more prevalent in **males (7:1)**, pyloric stenosis is the most common cause of acute bowel obstruction in children (affecting ~1 in 500 infants) and typically **presents between the 4th and 6th weeks of life**.

Diagnosis and investigation

> **Hx**
> - **Effortless, projectile** vomiting during or after feeds.
>   - The vomitus is ***never bilious***, although there may be small amounts of blood.
> - Depending on how long symptoms have been present, reduced fluid intake can lead to dry nappies and constipation.

Ex
- Assess the patient's growth (?small) and hydration status.
- Visible **peristaltic waves** in the upper quadrants of the abdomen (see *Fig. 9.11*), moving from left to right.
- A firm, mobile **'olive-sized' mass in the epigastrium**.

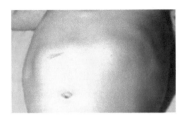
Fig. 9.11: Peristaltic wave in the left upper quadrant.

Ix
- Bloods: blood gases and U&Es will show **hypochloraemia**, **hypokalaemia** and **metabolic alkalosis**.
- An **abdominal USS** for diagnosis.

DDx
- GOR
- Overfeeding
- Duodenal atresia
- Gastroenteritis
- Food allergy

Management

- IV access should be gained and fluid resuscitation (if required) and maintenance therapy should be commenced. Fluid and metabolic derangements should be corrected before surgery.
- Definitive treatment is with a **Ramstedt's pyloromyotomy** – a longitudinal incision in the anterior wall of the pyloric canal to the level of the submucosa.

9.9.2 Appendicitis

Pathophysiology

- The appendix is a worm-like (vermiform) appendage of the caecum found in the right inguinal region; however, *in children, this anatomy may be different*.

Obstruction of the opening of the appendix, leading to stasis and subsequent bacterial overgrowth → Bacteria invade the wall of the appendix, which becomes inflamed → If left, the appendix may rupture, leading to **peritonitis**

Epidemiology and risk factors

- Appendicitis is the **most common cause of an acute abdomen** in children and affects up to ~10% of the population, typically from their early teenage years onwards.

Diagnosis and investigation

Hx
- Pain that begins around the **umbilicus before localizing to the right lower quadrant (RLQ)**.
- Patients are often **nauseous**.
- **Constipation** is common but, if there is rectal irritation, diarrhoea may be present.

Ex
- On inspection the patient may be lying still and will **look unwell**.
- Palpation of the abdomen will reveal tenderness in the RLQ – classically at **McBirney's Point** (⅓ distance between the anterior superior iliac spine and the umbilicus) – although in young children it may be poorly localized.
- **Rovsing's sign** – pain in the right iliac fossa when pressing in the left – may be present.

Ix
- No investigations are consistently helpful in diagnosis.
- Acute appendicitis is essentially a **clinical diagnosis**.
- As this can be difficult, children are often observed regularly to **look for progression** of the conditions.
- A urine dip and pregnancy test may be useful in excluding differentials.

DDx

APPENDICITIS:

Adenitis	**I**ntussusception
PID	**C**ystic ovaries
Pancreatitis	**I**BD
Ectopic pregnancy	**T**orsion of testes
Neoplasia	**I**BS
Diverticulitis	**S**tones

Management

- As treatment is surgical, the patient should be made **NBM and IV maintenance fluids** therefore started.
- **Analgesia** and **anti-emetics**.
- **Antibiotics** are started.
- **Surgical removal** is definitive.

OSCE tips 5: Peritonism

Irritation of the parietal peritoneum indicates significant pathology. On examination, these patients will have some typical features and it is important that you elicit these specifically:
- Rebound tenderness
- Involuntary guarding
- Pain with movement.

9.9.3 Mesenteric adenitis

Mesenteric adenitis (MA) is an important differential for acute appendicitis and RLQ pain in children.

Pathophysiology

- Symptoms are caused by inflammation of the mesenteric lymph nodes **secondary to a recent infection**, which causes a mild peritoneal irritation.

Epidemiology and risk factors

- Most common in children <15 years old.
- ≤20% of patients undergoing appendicectomy are found to have mesenteric adenitis.

Diagnosis and investigation

Diagnosis of mesenteric adenitis can only be confidently made in those who, at laparotomy/ laparoscopy, are found to have large mesenteric lymph nodes and whose appendix is normal.

Hx
- Abdominal pain in the **right lower quadrant**.
- The remaining symptoms are varied but can include:
  - fever
  - symptoms of an (URT) **infection** or tonsillitis.

Ex
- Patients *do not look as unwell* as those with appendicitis.
- **Fever is generally high**.
- The abdomen is tender, often in the RLQ, although it may be more diffuse.
  - There should be **no peritonism**.

Ix
This is a clinical diagnosis of exclusion. Investigations are therefore similar to those in acute appendicitis.

OSCE tips 6: Differentiating MA and appendicitis

	MA	Appendicitis
Temp (°C)	>38	37–38
Pharyngitis	+	–
Headache	+	–
Abdominal pain	+	+++
Involuntary guarding	–	+
Rebound tenderness	–	+
Shifting tenderness	+	Fixed
Vomiting	–	+/–

> **DDx** **APPENDICITIS**:
>
> | | |
> |---|---|
> | **A**ppendicitis | **I**ntussusception |
> | **P**ID | **C**ystic ovaries |
> | **P**ancreatitis | **I**BD |
> | **E**ctopic pregnancy | **T**orsion of testes |
> | **N**eoplasia | **I**BS |
> | **D**iverticulitis | **S**tones |

Management

- There is no specific management and symptoms are self-limiting.
- Analgesia is the mainstay; treat the causal infection if known.
- Due to diagnostic uncertainty, children are often admitted for a period of time for observation.

9.9.4 Intussusception

Intussusception is a telescoping of a proximal bowel segment into the immediately distal part (see *Fig. 9.12*).

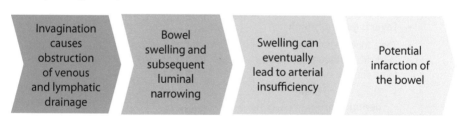

Fig. 9.12: Intussusception.

Pathophysiology

- The most common type is terminal **ileum into caecum (ileocaecal)**, but ileo–ileal and colocolic types also exist.
- The cause of the telescoping is usually **idiopathic (≥90%)**; however, in a small number of older children, there may be a pathological cause for this (i.e. Meckel diverticulum (75%), polyps/ Peutz–Jeghers syndrome, Henoch–Schönlein purpura).
- The pathological sequelae can be summarized as follows:

Invagination causes obstruction of venous and lymphatic drainage → Bowel swelling and subsequent luminal narrowing → Swelling can eventually lead to arterial insufficiency → Potential infarction of the bowel

Epidemiology and risk factors

- Intussusception is seen most often in children between the ages of 3 months and 2 years, peaking around 6–9 months.

Table 9.11: Risk factors for intussusception

Male sex (2–3:1)
Antecedent viral illness (weak)

Clinical features

Symptoms

- Colicky **abdominal pain** lasting for ~1–2 minutes is common.
  - The child typically screams and may bring their **knees to their chest**.
  - They are relatively asymptomatic between bouts (10–20 minutes).
- Per rectum bleeding, classically in the form of **'redcurrant jelly'**.
- **Early vomiting** that becomes bilious.

Signs

- Ensure baseline observations are stable: perforation rarely occurs, but can lead to sepsis and, on examination, peritonism.
- **Pallor** is common on inspection.
- Palpate the abdomen for a **'sausage-sized' mass in the right upper quadrant** (or epigastrium) and **empty RLQ** (Dance sign).

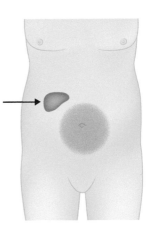

Fig. 9.13: The typical location of an abdominal mass (arrow) and distribution of abdominal pain (shaded).

Investigation and diagnosis

Hx
- Intermittent pain/crying, alongside bringing the knees to the chest.
- 'Redcurrant jelly' stools.
- Early, bilious vomit.

Ex
- Sausage-shaped mass ± Dance sign.
- If obstructed → distension.
- Assess for **peritonism**.

Ix
- Abdominal USS: target or doughnut sign – representing invagination of the bowel.
- AXR: gives a picture of bowel obstruction, with dilated bowel loops proximally and absence of gas distally. The leading edge of the obstruction typically has a 'rounded' appearance.
- **Contrast enema: gold standard** for diagnosis.

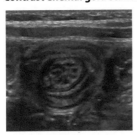

Fig. 9.14: The 'target sign' on USS.

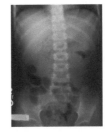

Fig. 9.15: Intussusception on plain AXR.

DDx	
• Cow's milk protein intolerance (→ bloody stools)	• Meckel diverticulum
• Hernia	• Appendicitis
• (Gastric) volvulus	• Gastroenteritis
	• Cyclical vomiting syndrome

Management

- As they are surgical patients, NBM and IV maintenance fluids are commenced.
- A nasogastric tube may be passed to decompress the stomach and bowel ('drip and suck').
- Analgesia and anti-emetics as required.

If **no signs** of peritonism, air (**or barium**) enema **is the treatment of choice.**

If signs of peritonism, this is a probable pathological lead point, or may indicate a failed enema. Surgical treatment with laparotomy is required.

9.9.5 Meckel diverticulum

Meckel diverticulum is a remnant of the vitellointestinal duct, an embryological structure that connects the midgut to the yolk sac. Importantly, it may contain aberrant tissue, typically gastric, pancreatic or jejunal.

Pathophysiology

Most remain asymptomatic throughout their lifetime (≥96%). Where symptoms do occur, they are principally through three mechanisms:

Haemorrhage
• This is primarily due to aberrant secretion of gastric acid, causing ulceration and subsequent bleeding in the adjacent ileum (not in the diverticulum itself, which is lined with gastric mucosa).

Obstruction
• A number of mechanisms are reported. The diverticulum may act as a fulcrum for volvulus formation, a lead point for intussusception or, due to recurrent inflammation, a stricture may form.

Inflammation (diverticulitis)
• Secondary to bacterial infection.

Epidemiology and risk factors

- The classical patient is a **toddler <2 y/o**; however, it may be seen in children up to 8 y/o.
- More common in males.

Clinical features

	Symptoms	Signs
Haemorrhage • Most common presentation in children	Bleeding per rectum, often substantial, which may be frank or mixed with stool	Check vital signs to ensure no haemodynamic compromise; otherwise essentially normal
Obstruction • Less common (25–40%) in children	(Absolute) constipation, absence of flatus, bilious vomiting and abdominal distension/tenderness	The abdomen will be distended and bowel sounds are classically 'tinkling' in obstruction in later stages
Inflammation • Predominantly seen in adults	Clinically similar to acute appendicitis, with pain originating in the periumbilical region and radiating to the RLQ	Similar to acute appendicitis, but tenderness is maximal periumbilically; there may be signs of peritonism

Investigation and diagnosis

Hx
- A toddler presenting, most commonly, with bleeding per rectum (PR); however, it is also an important differential in children with symptoms of obstruction or atypical features of acute appendicitis.

Ex
- Depending on presentation, it is important in the first instance to ensure that the child is not:
    - haemodynamically compromised: pale & clammy, cool peripherally, ↑HR ± ↓BP
    - peritonitic: involuntary guarding and rebound tenderness, typically periumbilically.
- Elicit signs of haemorrhage, obstruction or inflammation, as described above.

Ix
- Bloods: only necessary if bleeding PR. FBC will show ↓ Hb and haematocrit.
- Imaging:
    - Obstruction: **AXR** or CT – dilated bowel loops proximal to any obstruction.
    - Haemorrhage: **Technetium-99m pertechnetate scintigraphy** ('Meckel scan') is definitive in children presenting with PR bleeding, as it detects ectopic gastric mucosa in the diverticulum.

DDx
- **Haemorrhage:** IBD, infectious colitis, gastroenteritis, Peutz–Jeghers
- **Obstruction:** intussusception, Hirschsprung disease, volvulus
- **Inflammation:** acute appendicitis, IBD, IBS, Henoch–Schönlein purpura (HSP), constipation.

Management

- Definitive treatment is **surgical excision**; therefore the patient is NBM and has IV maintenance fluids commenced. Treat symptomatically before going to theatre.
- Adjunctive therapy is dependent on the complication:
  - If bleeding, a blood transfusion may be considered.
  - If obstructed, a nasogastric tube may be passed.

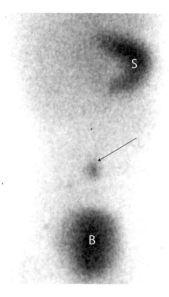

Fig. 9.16: A Meckel scan showing a diverticulum end on (arrow), along with uptake in the stomach (S) and bladder (B).

Chapter 10

Cardiovascular disorders

10.1 Acyanotic heart diseases

Pathophysiology

- The **majority of congenital defects are acyanotic**.
- They are typically broken down into **left-to-right shunts**, or **outflow obstruction**.

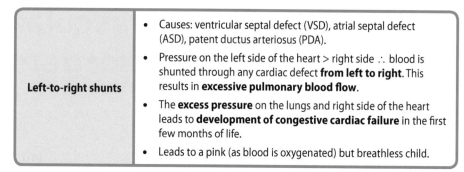

Left-to-right shunts	• Causes: ventricular septal defect (VSD), atrial septal defect (ASD), patent ductus arteriosus (PDA).
	• Pressure on the left side of the heart > right side ∴ blood is shunted through any cardiac defect **from left to right**. This results in **excessive pulmonary blood flow**.
	• The **excess pressure** on the lungs and right side of the heart leads to **development of congestive cardiac failure** in the first few months of life.
	• Leads to a pink (as blood is oxygenated) but breathless child.

Outflow obstruction	• Causes: aortic stenosis, pulmonary stenosis, coarctation of the aorta.
	• **Obstruction** in the **ventricular outflow tract** from either side of the heart results in **extra pressure** required to pump blood → **ventricular hypertrophy** and **insufficient cardiac output**.
	• Again, leads to a pink (as blood is oxygenated) but breathless child.

Clinical features

Table 10.1: Clinical features of left-to-right shunts

	Heart sounds	Surgical scars
VSD	Grade 3–6 pansystolic murmur	None (spontaneous closure) or median sternotomy
ASD	Fixed, split, loud S2 ± ejection systolic murmur over pulmonary area	Median sternotomy or no scar if closed via cardiac catheter
PDA (see *Chapter 3*)	Constant 'machinery' murmur through systole and diastole	Usually catheter closure via femoral route so no scar

Table 10.2: Clinical features of outflow obstruction

	Heart sounds	Surgical scars
Aortic stenosis	Loud ejection systolic murmur, loudest over aortic area	Nil, catheter repair via femoral route
Pulmonary stenosis (see *Section 10.3*)	Loud ejection systolic murmur, loudest over pulmonary area	Nil, balloon dilatation via femoral catheter
Coarctation of the aorta (see *Section 10.2*)	Weak or absent femoral pulses No murmur	Left thoracotomy

10.1.1 Ventricular septal defect

Pathophysiology

- Defect anywhere in ventricular septum → most commonly **perimembranous** (see *Fig. 10.1*).
- The amount of blood that moves across the defect depends on (a) the size and (b) the pulmonary vascular resistance (PVR).
- PVR is high at birth and drops over the first 2 months of life. As it decreases, the magnitude of the left-to-right shunt increases and this is why moderate–large VSDs present around 3 months of age with the infant in CHF.

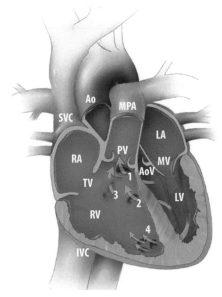

1. Conoventricular, Malaligned
2. Perimembranous
3. Inlet
4. Muscular

Fig. 10.1: Types of ventricular septal defect.
RA, right atrium; RV, right ventricle; LA, left atrium; LV, left ventricle; SVC, superior vena cava; IVC, inferior vena cava; MPA, main pulmonary artery; Ao, aorta.

Epidemiology and risk factors

30% of CHD, incidence 2:1000 live births; also often part of a more complex cardiac lesion.

Table 10.3: Risk factors for VSD	
• Trisomy 21	• Family history
• Presence of other cardiac lesions	• Maternal diabetes
	• Asian ethnicity

Diagnosis and investigation

Hx
- Antenatal or postnatal diagnosis?
- **Poor feeding** (sweaty, tachypnoeic and not able to finish feeds) suggests development of CHF.
- **Recurrent chest infection** in older children.

Ex
- **Pansystolic** murmur at left sternal edge.
- Smaller defect = louder murmur (greater turbulence which is what you are hearing). **N.B. very large defect may have no murmur**.
- Look for signs of **CHF** (tachycardia, tachypnoea, hepatomegaly).

Ix
- ECHO, ECG, CXR, oxygen saturations and 4 limb BP.

DDx
- Other CHD
- Lung disease
- PDA with large shunt

Management

- Small lesions (<3mm) will usually close spontaneously.
- **Large defects need surgical correction** → often with a patch. Without repair, large VSDs cause failure to thrive, heart failure and eventually **Eisenmenger syndrome** (see *Section 10.7*).
- Heart failure is managed with **diuretics**.
- Surgery generally performed at 3–6 months of age.

10.1.2 Atrial septal defect

Pathophysiology

Any defect in the atrial septum.
- Atrial septal defect (ASD) may be **primum** (10%, involving the endocardial cushions) or **secundum** (80%, affecting the middle portion of the septum).
- The defect causes **volume overload of the right side of the heart**, increasing pulmonary blood flow which, if untreated, causes **pulmonary hypertension**, **heart failure** and eventually **Eisenmenger syndrome**.

Epidemiology and risk factors

- Accounts for **5%** of congenital heart disease.

Table 10.4: Risk factors for ASD
Female sex (2:1 F:M)
Maternal alcohol intake in pregnancy
Family history

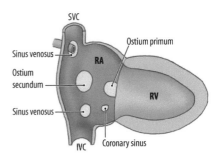

Fig. 10.2: Location of the types of ASD as viewed from the right atrium.
IVC, inferior vena cava; RA, right atrium; RV, right ventricle; SVC, superior vena cava; TV, tricuspid valve; MV, mitral valve; PV, pulmonary valve; AoV, aortic valve.

Diagnosis and investigation

Hx
- Usually **asymptomatic** with no signs or symptoms before 3–4 years of age.
- Older children may present with recurrent **infections** or, very rarely, CHF.
- In adulthood presentation is with development of **pulmonary hypertension** and **heart failure** or **arrhythmias** (from progressive right-sided cardiac dilatation affecting conduction system) in the 3rd or 4th decade of life.

Ex
- Ejection systolic murmur loudest in pulmonary area (**increased flow through pulmonary valve**) and **fixed split S2** because of constant right-side **volume overload**.
- Signs of **CHF** (tachycardia, tachypnoea, hepatomegaly, failure to thrive) may be present in an older child with a large unrepaired ASD.

Ix
- **Echocardiogram** – to assess size of defect and amount of pulmonary blood flow.
- **CXR** – variable cardiomegaly, increased vascular markings.
- **ECG** – right axis deviation, right bundle branch block (RBBB), right ventricular hypertrophy (RVH).

DDx
- VSD
- Complete atrioventricular septal defect (AVSD)
- Complex cardiac defect
- Idiopathic pulmonary hypertension

Management

- **Small defects** (3–8mm) usually close **spontaneously** by 18 months of age.
- **Larger defects (>8mm)** need surgical management or, more commonly now, closure via cardiac catheter.
- All **primum defects** that do not spontaneously resolve need **surgical closure**.
- Congestive cardiac failure is managed with diuretics.

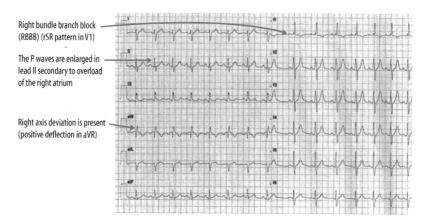

Right bundle branch block (RBBB) (rSR pattern in V1)

The P waves are enlarged in lead II secondary to overload of the right atrium

Right axis deviation is present (positive deflection in aVR)

Fig. 10.3: ECG in a 4-year-old with an ASD.

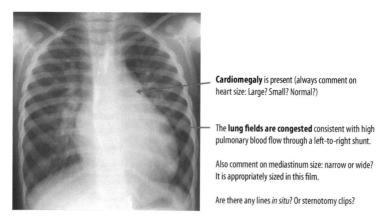

Cardiomegaly is present (always comment on heart size: Large? Small? Normal?)

The **lung fields are congested** consistent with high pulmonary blood flow through a left-to-right shunt.

Also comment on mediastinum size: narrow or wide? It is appropriately sized in this film.

Are there any lines *in situ*? Or sternotomy clips?

Fig. 10.4: Chest X-ray of a child with an unrepaired VSD.

OSCE tips 1: The paediatric cardiovascular exam

- **Be prepared** for a cardiac child in your OSCE – there are a lot of them and post-repair they are typically stable with good signs, so are frequently used in exams.
- **Comment on appearance** – are they pale? Are they blue? Are they clubbed? Well grown or small? Dysmorphic? Can you see a sternotomy from the end of the bed?
- **Pulses – make a point of checking for the femorals and commenting.** We do **brachial (not radial)** pulse checks in babies – if you check a baby's radial pulse in your OSCE it will be clear to the examiner you have not examined many paediatric patients.
- Check for posterior thoracotomy **scars.**
- **Listen, then listen again, then once more.** If you hear a murmur be specific. If you don't, be confident. Even if there is no murmur, are the heart sounds normal?
- **Practise, practise, practise.** Children, especially babies, breathe fast and at first it is easy to mistake breath sounds for a murmur. Only by listening to normal hearts and chests will you be able to identify an abnormality.

Pathophysiology

Narrowing of the thoracic aorta, usually where the ductus arteriosus originates from.	Exact mechanism unclear. Ranges in severity from mild narrowing to total interruption of the aortic arch.	A severe coarctation will result in **circulatory collapse with weak/absent femoral pulses** soon after birth.	Less severe coarctations present later in life with **systemic hypertension**.

Epidemiology and risk factors

- 8–10% of congenital heart disease.
- 4 in 10 000 live births.

Table 10.5: Risk factors for coarctation

Male sex (2:1 M:F)
Turner syndrome (45,X)

Investigation and diagnosis

Hx
- Severity-dependent. **Interrupted** or **severely narrowed arches** present with **neonatal collapse** in the first few days of life, as the ductus arteriosus closes.
- Less severe cases are picked up incidentally when **hypertension** is noticed or if the child has symptomatic hypertension (headaches, visual changes, renal impairment).

Ex
- Hallmark examination findings of CoA:
  - **differential blood pressure** – higher in the arm than the leg
  - **absent/weak/delayed femoral pulses** – you must always comment on an infant's femoral pulses during a cardiovascular examination.
- **A murmur is atypical** and more likely to reflect **stenosis of a bicuspid aortic valve**.

Ix
- **CXR – cardiomegaly**, increased vascular markings, **rib notching** >5 y/o (from collateral vessel development eroding part of the rib).
- **ECG** – may be normal, show RBBB or RVH. In older children who have developed systemic hypertension, left ventricular hypertrophy is common.
- **Echocardiogram** – diagnostic. Allows assessment of exact anatomy and other defects.

DDx
- Hypovolaemia (of any cause)
- Heart failure (any cause)
- Complex congenital heart disease

Management

- **Symptomatic neonate**: prostaglandin E1 (prostin) to maintain patent ductus arteriosus, treat hypertension and urgent surgical repair.
- **Asymptomatic children**: surgery indicated in hypertension, CHF or collateral blood vessel formation. Medically manage hypertension. Closely monitor for secondary organ damage.

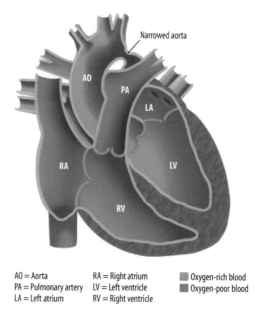

AO = Aorta	RA = Right atrium	▨ Oxygen-rich blood
PA = Pulmonary artery	LV = Left ventricle	▨ Oxygen-poor blood
LA = Left atrium	RV = Right ventricle	

Fig. 10.5: Coarctation of the aorta.

Pulmonary stenosis

Pathophysiology

Any lesion that **restricts outflow** through the pulmonary area. May be **valvular** (90%; usually due to partial fusion or thickening of the valve leaflets), **subvalvular** (seen in tetralogy of Fallot (TOF)) or **supravalvular**. **Right ventricular hypertrophy** and **heart failure** develop: this is proportional to the degree of stenosis.

Epidemiology and risk factors

- Accounts for **8%** of congenital heart disease.
- A dysplastic, thickened valve is frequently seen in **Noonan syndrome**.

Table 10.6: Risk factors for pulmonary stenosis
• Family history
• Tetralogy of Fallot
• Noonan syndrome

Diagnosis and investigation

Hx
- Usually **asymptomatic**.
- If stenosis is critical, it will present in the neonatal period with cyanosis and circulatory collapse.
- Older children with moderate stenosis develop **exertional dyspnoea** and **fatigue** easily, similar to aortic stenosis.
- Severe stenosis will result in **heart failure**.

Ex
- Auscultation reveals a **widely split S2** and, if valvular, there will be an ejection **'click'**. An **ejection systolic murmur** is heard over the pulmonary area and **radiates to the back**.
- **Critical stenosis** has a quiet or absent murmur in an unwell, cyanosed infant.

Ix
- **ECG** (may show RVH and/or RAD).
- **Echocardiogram**.
- **Chest X-ray** will typically show a prominent pulmonary artery.

DDx
- Critical pulmonary stenosis
- Tetralogy of Fallot
- Aortic stenosis

Management

- *Critical* pulmonary stenosis in the neonate is an indication for **prostaglandin infusion** and urgent transfer to a cardiac centre.
- **Balloon valvuloplasty** ('dilatation'; *Fig. 10.6*) is performed in severe or symptomatic stenosis.
- **Surgery** is indicated in subvalvular stenosis or for those with valvular stenosis resistant to balloon dilatation.

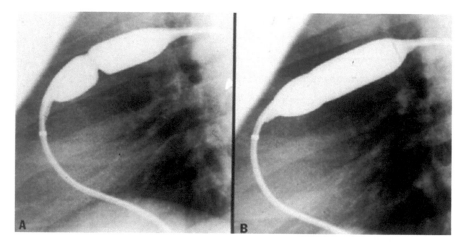

Fig. 10.6: A stenotic pulmonary valve before (A) and after (B) balloon dilatation.

Cyanotic heart diseases

Cyanotic cardiac defects occur if **sufficient** <u>**deoxygenated**</u> **blood enters the systemic circulation**. This may be because **flow to the lungs is obstructed**, or because **blood is being shunted from right to left** ∴ bypassing the pulmonary circulation.

Pathophysiology

Right-to-left shunts

- Causes: transposition of the great arteries, tetralogy of Fallot (TOF).
- If sufficient deoxygenated blood enters the systemic circulation via any defect the child will be cyanosed, **typically visible** once saturations drop to **≤85%**.
- If there is **decreased pulmonary blood flow** the child will **not be breathless** (i.e. TOF or any major right-sided obstruction (such as tricuspid or pulmonary atresia)).

Mixed shunt

- Causes: AVSD, truncus arteriosus.
- **Intracardiac mixing** of oxygenated and deoxygenated blood results in a **milder cyanosis**.
- Blood preferentially flows from left to right, so increasing pulmonary blood flow, resulting in a child both **blue** (due to mixing) <u>**and breathless**</u> (due to increased pulmonary flow).

Outflow obstruction

- Causes: hypoplastic left heart, interrupted aortic arch.
- These lesions are rarer and the child has **'duct-dependent' circulation,** meaning all the blood to the pulmonary or systemic circulation (depending on where the lesion is) is via the ductus arteriosus. **When the ductus arteriosus closes the child will present in circulatory collapse** → shock, acidosis and sometimes death.
- Presentation is **typically day 2–3 of life**, as the duct closes at this time.

Clinical features and sequelae of cyanosis

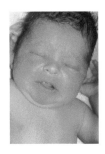

- **Cyanosis** appears as a blue discoloration or hue of the mucous membranes, lips, tongue, nailbeds ± skin.
- **Digital clubbing** – exact mechanism is unclear. Develops after around 6 months of age.
- **Hypoxic 'tet' spells** – see the end of *Section 10.4.1* for a full description. It can be seen in any cyanotic condition and severe spells may result in death.

Fig. 10.7: Cyanosis in a newborn. Note the subtle blue discoloration around the mouth.

- **Polycythaemia** – low arterial oxygen saturations **stimulate EPO** production from the **kidneys** → **increase RBC production from the bone marrow.** Whilst this increases oxygen-carrying capacity, it also **increases blood viscosity** ∴ ↑ **risk of thromboembolic events.**

OSCE tips 2: Digital clubbing in children

Clubbing in children is uncommon, except in certain conditions, which include:
- Cardiac disease
- Pulmonary disease, especially cystic fibrosis
- Tuberculosis
- GI diseases, such as Crohn's, UC and coeliac disease.

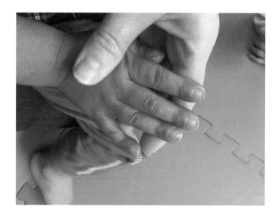

Fig. 10.8: Digital clubbing and cyanosis in a child with congenital heart disease.

10.4.1 Tetralogy of Fallot

Pathophysiology

A collection of **four abnormalities:**

Epidemiology and risk factors

The **most common** of the cyanotic lesions. 10% of CHD (around 1 in 2500 births). Most cases are sporadic.

Features of TOF

1. **Large VSD**

2. **Overriding aorta**

3. **Pulmonary stenosis causing right ventricular (RV) outflow obstruction**

4. **RV hypertrophy secondary to RV outflow obstruction**

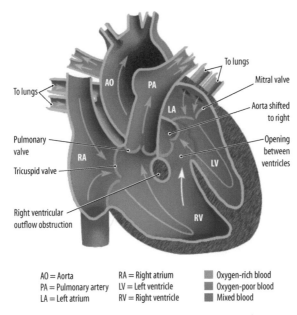

AO = Aorta   RA = Right atrium   ■ Oxygen-rich blood
PA = Pulmonary artery   LV = Left ventricle   ■ Oxygen-poor blood
LA = Left atrium   RV = Right ventricle   ■ Mixed blood

Fig. 10.9: Congenital defects, and subsequent blood flow, in tetralogy of Fallot.

Table 10.7: Risk factors for TOF	
• Rubella in pregnancy • Maternal age >40 • Family history	• Maternal diabetes • Maternal poor nutrition or alcohol intake during pregnancy

Diagnosis and investigation

Hx
- **Variable** from a very sick neonate at birth with severe cyanosis to an asymptomatic acyanotic child.
- **Older children** that have not undergone repair will have **dyspnoea on exertion** and there will be a history of **'tet spells'**. Those acyanotic at birth tend to become blue by 3 years of age.

Ex
- Variably cyanotic.
- Loud **ejection systolic murmur** due to pulmonary stenosis NOT the VSD.
- **S2 is loud** ± palpable thrill.

Ix
- **Echocardiogram** is diagnostic.
- **ECG** shows right axis deviation and RV hypertrophy.
- **CXR** shows a **'boot-shaped' heart**.

Management

General management:

- Surgical repair is typically performed around 6 months of age.
- Manage CHF and iron deficiency if present.

Tet spell management:

- Tet spells occur when the child has an acute drop in pulmonary blood flow, making them acutely hypoxic, usually after an episode of rapid breathing and crying.
- **Hold child knee-to-chest** (to increase venous return). Give small morphine dose to settle rapid breathing and relax ventricular outflow tract. Occasionally propranolol is needed.

10.4.2 Transposition of the great arteries (TGA)

Pathophysiology

The aorta arises from the right ventricle and the pulmonary artery from the left ventricle, leaving the infant with two entirely separate circulations (*Fig. 10.10*). Consequently there is an associated VSD/ASD or PDA to allow some mixing of the two systems.

Without this, the child will present quickly with circulatory collapse, acidosis and death.

Epidemiology and risk factors

5% of CHD (1 in 5000 live births).

Table 10.8: Risk factors for TGA
Male sex (3:1)
Maternal diabetes

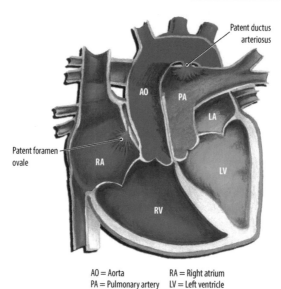

AO = Aorta	RA = Right atrium
PA = Pulmonary artery	LV = Left ventricle
LA = Left atrium	RV = Right ventricle

Fig. 10.10: Transposition of the great arteries.

Diagnosis and investigation

Hx
- Cyanosed from birth with **rapidly developing heart failure**.
- May have been **antenatally diagnosed** on ultrasound.

Ex
- **Unwell** neonate, tachypnoeic, tachycardic, **cyanotic** and often hypoglycaemic.
- There will be **no murmur, unless there is a VSD** (40% of cases). **S2 is loud and single**.
- Signs of heart failure (oedema, hepatomegaly).

Ix
- ECG: RAD and RVH.
- Echocardiogram.
- CXR (cardiomegaly, 'egg-on-a-string' shape is characteristic).

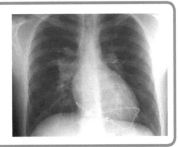

Fig. 10.11: CXR demonstrating 'egg-on-a-string' appearance of the cardiac silhouette.

DDx
- Persistent pulmonary hypertension of the newborn
- Other cyanotic heart diseases

Management

1. **Prostaglandin** infusion (to maintain PDA).
2. Urgent **transfer to cardiac centre**.
3. Those without a VSD require urgent intervention with a **balloon septostomy** to allow mixing of the two circulatory systems.
4. CHF is managed with **diuretics**.
5. Surgery is performed at 3 weeks of age (**arterial switch procedure**).

OSCE tips 3: TGA prognosis

TGA is rarely associated with other defects so following repair these children often do very well, and the only evidence of prior illness is their sternotomy scar. Long-term survival is approximately 95%.

10.4.3 Univentricular circulations

Pathophysiology

Hypoplastic left heart syndrome (HLHS)

HLHS results from insufficient development of the left ventricle, which is very small. The aortic and mitral valves are small or absent.

An ASD is required to permit mixing of oxygenated and deoxygenated blood, reaching the systemic circulation via a patent ductus arteriosus.

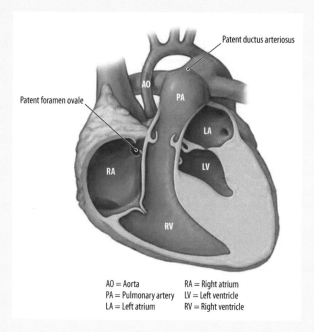

AO = Aorta   RA = Right atrium
PA = Pulmonary artery   LV = Left ventricle
LA = Left atrium   RV = Right ventricle

Fig. 10.12: Hypoplastic left heart syndrome (HLHS) – note the ASD and large ductus arteriosus.

Tricuspid atresia

In tricuspid atresia, a similar situation arises on the right side of the heart. Absence of the tricuspid valve causes hypoplasia of the right ventricle.

Blood reaches the left side of the heart via an ASD, and is then pumped to the pulmonary circulation via a VSD.

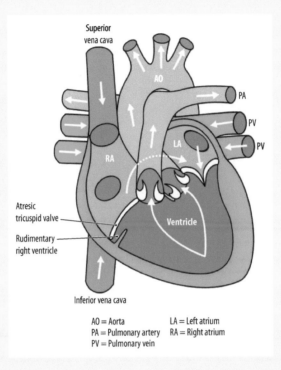

AO = Aorta   LA = Left atrium
PA = Pulmonary artery   RA = Right atrium
PV = Pulmonary vein

Fig. 10.13: Tricuspid atresia. Note the rudimentary, hypoplastic right ventricle and how the blood from the right atrium reaches the ventricles via an ASD (dotted arrow). The colour of the blood indicates its degree of oxygenation.

Management

The aim with all children with univentricular circulation is to palliate them (as none of these lesions can be cured) with a series of surgeries that aim to have the **well-developed ventricle provide systemic circulation**, and to have the body's **systemic venous return drain directly to the pulmonary arteries**, bypassing the heart altogether.

This is typically done over **2–3 surgeries in the first 2–3 years of life**. Once this has been achieved the child is described as having a **'Fontan circulation'**.

10.5 Cardiac infections

10.5.1 Infective endocarditis (IE)

Pathophysiology

Structural abnormalities causing **turbulent blood flow** disrupt the cardiac **endothelium**, making it susceptible to **bacterial adherence**, where even transient bacteraemia may progress to infective endocarditis. Organisims isolated are typically *Streptococcus viridans* (α-haemolytic strep), *Staphylococcus aureus* and enterococci (γ-haemolytic).

Epidemiology and risk factors

Affects **0.5:1000**. Most children have underlying structural heart disease.

Table 10.9: Risk factors for endocarditis

• Congenital heart disease	• Valve prosthesis
	• Bacteraemia
• Previous endocarditis	

Diagnosis and investigation

Hx Variable presentation. May be non-specifically unwell with fever of unknown origin. May present with sequelae of septic emboli (strokes, seizures).

Ex Obs may be normal or in keeping with sepsis, **low grade fever** typical. New **murmur** is typical and present in most cases. **Splenomegaly** is common. Look for peripheral vascular and immunological phenomena (see Duke's minor criteria). Note: these are more common in adults than children with IE.

Ix Serial blood cultures, ECHO, FBC, ESR.
Diagnosis made with **Duke's criteria** (overleaf), **which is positive if there are**:
- 2 major criteria OR
- 1 major + 3 minor OR
- No major + 5 minor.

DDx
- Other causes of infection
- Previously undiagnosed structural heart disease

Duke's major criteria	Duke's minor criteria
1. Two positive blood cultures with a typical IE organism. 2. Echocardiogram findings consistent with IE (new valve regurgitation, new mass or abscess, dehiscence of prosthetic valve).	1. Predisposing heart defect. 2. **Vascular** phenomena (arterial emboli, septic pulmonary infarcts, Janeway lesions, conjunctival haemorrhage). 3. **Immunological** phenomena (glomerulonephritis, Osler nodes, Roth spots). 4. Fever >38°C. 5. Positive blood cultures that do not fit major criteria.

Management

- **4–6 weeks of IV antibiotics** targeted to causative organism; needs discussion with microbiologist.
- If prosthetic valve infected it must usually be removed because it is very difficult to eradicate infection from prosthetic material.
- Fungal endocarditis is treated with amphotericin B; it is associated with poor prognosis.

OSCE tips 4: Antibiotics and dental procedures

Antibiotic prophylaxis is no longer indicated before dental or surgical procedures but you need to be aware that any child with CHD is at an increased risk of endocarditis (NICE 2016 guidelines).

10.5.2 Pericarditis

Pathophysiology

Pericarditis is inflammation of the pericardial sac, usually due to viral infection. Other causes include bacterial infection or systemic inflammatory disease (such as systemic lupus erythematosus (SLE)).

Epidemiology and risk factors

In infants, viral illness is the most common cause; outside the UK rheumatic fever is a well-recognized cause. May also complicate TB, cardiac surgery, oncology treatment or as part of a wider inflammatory arthritis.

Table 10.10: Risk factors for pericarditis

• Rheumatic fever	• Cardiac surgery
• Viral illness	• Inflammatory arthritis

Diagnosis and investigation

Hx Stabbing or aching central **chest pain**, may radiate to head/neck, typically **worse on inspiration** and **lying down**.

May progress to cardiac tamponade causing acute circulatory collapse

Ex May be **tachycardic, tachypnoeic** and **pyrexial**. Auscultate for **pericardial friction rub**. Look for signs of cardiac tamponade (pulsus paradoxus, **quiet heart sounds**, distended neck veins).

Ix ECG, ECHO (to assess pericardial effusion), CXR (enlarged heart). **Pericardiocentesis** may be utilized to identify the cause.

DDx
- MI
- PE
- Aortic dissection
- Angina
- Coronary artery spasm
- GORD
- Oesophageal spasm

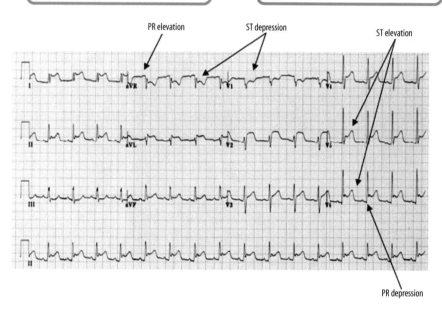

Fig. 10.14: ECG showing findings in pericarditis, with **ST elevation** (characteristically described as 'saddle-shaped') and **PR depression** the *most typical*.

Management

- **Urgent decompression of any tamponade**.
- Viral pericarditis managed conservatively.
- Purulent bacterial pericarditis needs IV antibiotics for 4–6 weeks.
- **Constrictive pericarditis** requires complete **resection of the pericardium**.

Cardiac arrhythmias

In children, sinus arrhythmia (variation of the heart rate with breathing) is normal. The **most common symptomatic arrhythmia in children is supraventricular tachycardia** (SVT) but arrhythmias should be considered in all children with syncope, palpitations or chest pain. Note that most children with palpitations do not have a pathological arrhythmia.

10.6.1 Supraventricular tachycardia

Pathophysiology

Narrow complex tachycardia usually >220bpm, usually from activation of a secondary pathway causing a re-entry tachycardia through the AV node.

Epidemiology and risk factors

Around half of children with SVT will have no underlying heart disease; 10–20% will have Wolff–Parkinson–White syndrome (WPW).

Table 10.11: Risk factors for SVT

* Structural heart disease
* WPW
* Following cardiac surgery

Diagnosis and investigation

Hx May be asymptomatic. **Palpitations** and **dizziness**, presyncope, **syncope**. May complain of chest pain during episodes.

Ix **ECG:** shows narrow complex tachycardia with no visible P waves.
Bloods (electrolytes, infection markers).

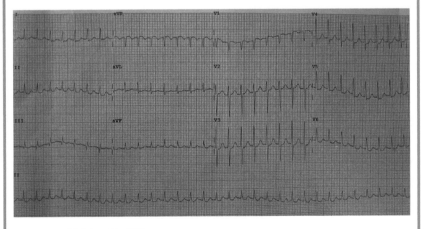

Fig. 10.15: ECG showing SVT.

> **Ex**   **Tachycardic.** May look well or shocked: with haemodynamic compromise (↓ BP, ↑ CRT, ↑ RR) and signs of heart failure.
> Ask about feeding and irritability in younger children.

> **DDx**
> - Atrial fibrillation
> - Atrial flutter
> - Ventricular tachycardia
> - Sinus arrhythmia

Management

| Haemodynamically **STABLE** | ABCDE. Attach high flow oxygen and cardiac monitor. Obtain IV access. | Vagal manoeuvres | Adenosine IV 50mcg/kg up to 12mg max. |

| Haemodynamically **UNSTABLE** | ABDCE and call for urgent senior help. Attach high flow oxygen and cardiac monitor. Get best IV access possible. | Synchronized cardioversion 0.5J/kg up to 2J per kg. |

10.6.2 Long QT syndrome

Pathophysiology

Disorder of ventricular repolarization, such that the time for the ventricles to repolarize is increased. These children are at increased risk of **life-threatening arrhythmias** (ventricular tachycardia and torsades de pointes (TdP)) and **sudden cardiac death**. **Normal QT is <440ms.**

Epidemiology and risk factors

Consider in all children with **syncope**, especially episodes brought on by **stress, emotion** or **exercise**. There are **congenital** forms (secondary to ion channel mutations) and **acquired** (drugs, electrolyte imbalance).

Table 10.12: Risk factors for long QT	
• Cardiac ion channel mutation • Cardiomyopathy	• Family history • QT-prolonging drugs

Diagnosis and investigation

Hx — Range from asymptomatic to presyncope, **palpitations**, syncope, **seizures** or **cardiac arrest**. Ask about **family history** (positive in 60%) of sudden cardiac death/unexplained death in a young person. **Syncope triggered by stress, loud noises** or exercise (particularly **swimming**) should raise suspicion of long QT.

Ex — Likely normal. **Autosomal recessive** inherited long QT syndromes are associated with **congenital deafness**.

Ix — **ECG**. Electrolytes (**magnesium** and **potassium** especially). ECHO for structural defects. Consider testing for ion channel mutations.

DDx —
• Transient long QT secondary to medication
• Other arrhythmia

OSCE tips 5: Calculating QTc

The QT interval is inversely correlated with the heart rate: as HR increases, the QT interval shortens.

It is necessary, therefore, to 'correct' the QT interval, to calculate it at a HR of 60 (QTc).

$$QTc = QT\,interval/\sqrt{(RR\,interval)}$$

Management`

- **Avoid** QT-prolonging drugs.
- Avoid **competitive sports** and **swimming**.
- **Beta-blockers** (which reduce syncope and risk of sudden cardiac death) should be given to all symptomatic children.

- An **implantable cardioverter defibrillator** (ICD) for high-risk patients (those with previous cardiac arrest or still having cardiac events despite beta-blockers; or if QTc is >600ms).
- Acquired long QT – treat electrolyte abnormality and stop QT-prolonging drugs.

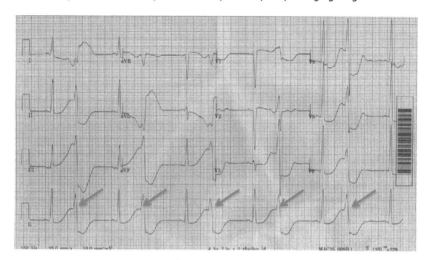

Fig. 10.16: ECG showing a **QTc of >600ms**. There are ventricular **ectopics** falling on every late **T wave** (blue arrows) putting this patient at very high risk of developing TdP rhythm. This is best appreciated in the rhythm strip (lead II).

Pulmonary hypertension

Defined as a **mean pulmonary artery pressure gradient >25mmHg at rest**. This section focuses on the physiology and management of cardiac causes.

Pathophysiology

Left-to-right shunt	• Such as a VSD, ASD or PDA results in **high pulmonary blood flow**, increasing pulmonary pressure.

Remodelling	• Over time **remodelling** of the **pulmonary vasculature** occurs and it becomes **permanently and irreversibly constricted, further increasing pressure**. • High pulmonary pressure causes **right ventricular hypertrophy** and **right-sided heart failure**.

Shunt reversal	• When the pressure in the lungs reaches a critical level, the original left-to-right **shunt reverses** and **Eisenmenger syndrome** has developed. • Prognosis at this point is very poor and life expectancy is a few years without heart–lung transplant.

Epidemiology and risk factors

Epidemiology depends on the underlying cause.

Diagnosis and investigation

Table 10.13: Risk factors for pulmonary hypertension

• CHD
• Chronic lung disease
• Obstructive sleep apnoea

Hx
- **Progressive breathlessness**, fatigue, reduced exercise tolerance.
- Presyncope, **chest pain** or **syncope on exertion**.
- Asymptomatic in earlier stages.

Ex
- May be **cyanotic** and **tachypnoeic**.
- **S2 is loud**; **diastolic murmur** of pulmonary regurgitation is common.
- Signs of right-sided heart failure (**hepatomegaly** and **peripheral oedema**).
- Examine for **clubbing** and surgical scars.

Ix
- ECG, CXR, ECHO, cardiac catheter (to confirm diagnosis)

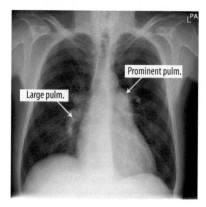

Fig. 10.17: A chest X-ray showing typical features of pulmonary hypertension.

DDx Underlying cause:
- PE
- Lung disease
- Heart disease
- Inflammatory disease
- Idiopathic

Management

- **Remove** or treat **underlying cause**. Until vascular remodelling occurs the process is reversible so **early identification and treatment are key**.
- Heart failure is managed with **diuretics**.
- **Pulmonary vasodilators** (sildenafil) are given if vascular remodelling has not yet occurred (ineffective after this).

Chapter 11

Renal and genitourinary disorders

Congenital abnormalities

There is a wide spectrum of congenital renal tract abnormalities – sometimes seen as part of a multisystem disorder – which vary from incidental findings to fatal conditions.

Pathophysiology

Defect	Embryology	Incidence	Management
Renal agenesis	Total absence of one or both kidneys	1:4000 (bilateral) 1:3000 (unilateral)	Fatal if bilateral A normal single kidney has good prognosis, but the child will need monitoring for complications
Multicystic dysplastic kidney	The renal cortex is replaced with multiple cysts, leaving no functioning cortex	1:2000–4000	Fatal if bilateral If unilateral, close monitoring for complications → nephrectomy if these develop and are not responsive to medical therapy
Horseshoe kidney	Fusion of the inferior poles of the 2 kidneys across the midline Both function independently	1:500	Generally asymptomatic, but at higher risk of renal/urological complications than a normal kidney Treat these as needed
Duplex kidney	A single kidney has 2 separate pelvicalyceal systems	1:100–200	Generally asymptomatic, but at higher risk of renal/urological complications than a normal kidney Treat these as needed
Posterior urethral valves	Urethral obstruction from a valve-like fold of tissue	1:50 000 (males only)	Dependent on the degree of obstruction Surgical management is definitive
Autosomal dominant polycystic kidney disease	Multiple, progressive cyst formation within the kidneys	1:1000	Progressive disease, which leads to dialysis in ~50% of patients (by ~60 years of age), initial treatment is management of complications
Pelviureteric junction obstruction	Inadequate canalization of the pelviureteric junction, leading to obstruction	1:1000	Often requires no treatment If complications develop, surgical management may be required

Epidemiology and risk factors

- Occurs in 1 in 200–400 live births.
- More common in males.
- Higher incidence in the context of multi-system disorders and syndromes.

Table 11.1: Risk factors for renal tract defects

Family history
Maternal diabetes
Male sex
Turner syndrome (45,X)

Investigation and diagnosis

Hx
- Maternal oligohydramnios (amniotic fluid produced by foetal micturition)
- Family history of renal disease
- Ask about UTIs in older children

Ex
- If there has been oligohydramnios, there are likely to be respiratory issues
- Thorough examination for other anomalies and dysmorphic facies (?related to a syndrome)
- Palpate abdomen for renal masses

Ix
- **USS** – for anatomy, assess for hydronephrosis/hydroureter. Does not describe function.
- **MCUG** – micturating cystourogram. Contrast instilled into bladder via catheter to assess for retrograde flow of urine (vesicoureteric reflux; VUR) and ureteric obstruction.
- **DMSA** – static nuclear scan of the renal cortex, picks up functional defects (scars).
- **MAG 3** – dynamic nuclear scan, measures urinary drainage, used to pick up VUR in older children by performing scan during micturition.
- **Urine dip** – for haematuria, proteinuria and markers of infection.
- **U&Es** – for renal function (be aware children don't achieve best renal function until over 2 years of age).

DDx Isolated renal tract anomaly or part of a systemic condition?

OSCE tips: Potter syndrome

Anomalies resulting in little/no foetal urine (i.e. bilateral renal agenesis, multicystic dysplastic kidneys) cause oligohydramnios. This leads to foetal compression and produces a constellation of features known as Potter syndrome:
- Pulmonary hypoplasia
- Potter facies (prominent infraorbital folds, low-set ears, micrognathia, beaked nose with flat nasal bridge) – see *Fig. 11.1.*
- Club foot or other lower limb anomalies.

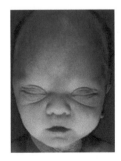

Fig. 11.1: Typical facies of Potter syndrome.

11.2 Urinary tract infection

Urinary tract infection (UTI) – a common problem. Prompt diagnosis and treatment are crucial to avoid damage to the upper renal tract, which can result in scarring, chronic renal failure and hypertension.

Pathophysiology

Although UTIs may affect children without any predisposition, it is important to consider structural anomalies as the aetiology. The most common organism is *Escherichia coli* (↑*Pseudomonas* spp. in children with structural disease).

Epidemiology and risk factors

- 1% of boys and 3% of girls will develop a UTI before the age of 11.
- **Half of children with a UTI have a structural defect** of the urinary tract.

Table 11.2: Risk factors for UTI	
Female sex	• Shorter urethra predisposes to infection
Structural defect in the urinary tract	• Stagnation of urine predisposes to infection
Vesicoureteric reflux (VUR)	• Causes ureteric dilatation and incomplete voiding; see *Fig. 11.2*
Incomplete bladder emptying	• Stagnation of urine allows bacteria to replicate and cause infection
Constipation	• Puts pressure on bladder and may cause incomplete emptying

Clinical features

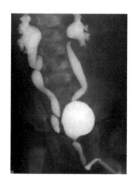

Symptoms
- Older children → dysuria, frequency, abdominal (especially loin) pain
- Vomiting
- Young babies and neonates → lethargy and irritability.

Signs
- Fever
- Poor feeding and vomiting (may be the only signs in a neonate)
- Jaundice (especially in neonates)
- Sepsis (SIRS response with deranged observations).

Fig. 11.2: MCUG showing bilateral VUR.

Investigation and diagnosis

Hx
- Age dependent.
- High index of suspicion in younger children is needed. Poor feeding, vomiting, irritability.
- In older children loin pain, dysuria and frequency.

Ix
- Urine dip, **urine for MC&S**.
- **Bloods** (FBC, U&Es, ↑ CRP) and **blood cultures**.
- **Ultrasound** (to identify pyelonephritis and structural defects) and **other imaging** – see NICE guidance in *Table 11.3*.

Ex
- Observations may be stable or reflect sepsis ± fever.
- Palpate for abdominal masses and tenderness.

DDx
- Sepsis of other origin
- Vesicoureteric reflux
- Vulvitis
- Balanitis

Table 11.3: NICE guidelines (2017) for imaging in children <6 months old with UTI

Test	Responds well to treatment within 48 hours	Atypical UTI[a]	Recurrent UTI[a]
Ultrasound during the acute infection	No	Yes[c]	Yes
Ultrasound within 6 weeks	Yes[b]	No	No
DMSA 4–6 months following the acute infection	No	Yes	Yes
MCUG	No	Yes	Yes

[a]Septic or seriously ill, poor urine flow, abdominal mass, raised creatinine, failure to respond to antibiotics within 48 hours, non-*E. coli* organism. Recurrent if 3 or more lower tract infections; 2 or more upper tract infections.
[b]If abnormal consider MCUG.
[c]In an infant or child with a non-*E. coli* UTI, responding well to antibiotics and with no other features of atypical infection, the ultrasound can be requested on a non-urgent basis to take place within 6 weeks.

Management

- **Antibiotics** – initially empirical and then guided by MC&S results.
- Antipyretics for fever and analgesia for pain.
- **Long-term management:**
  - Prophylactic antibiotics are sometimes used in children with recurrent UTIs (especially if <2 years of age) and those with severe VUR.
  - **Preventative measures** – encourage high oral fluid intake, regular voiding and good hygiene. Treat constipation if present.

Renal damage due to **retrograde flow of urine** from the bladder → upper renal tract. This may be due to **incompetence at the vesicoureteric junction** (common), secondary to obstruction (i.e. posterior urethral valve) or a neurogenic bladder (that fails to void adequately).

Pathophysiology

Reflux of urine → recurrent upper tract infection → scarring (nephropathy) → HTN + CKD

Epidemiology and risk factors

- Seen in 1% of children.
- 30–50% of children with vesicoureteric reflux have a first-degree relative with the condition.

Table 11.4: Risk factors for reflux nephropathy

Family history
Recurrent UTIs
Anatomical renal tract abnormality

Diagnosis and investigation

Hx
- May be **asymptomatic** or present with **recurrent UTIs**.
- Ask about **family history**.

Ex
- Observations:
  - Assess for hypertension
  - Features of UTI/sepsis?
- Palpate the abdomen
  - Loin pain?
  - Enlarged kidneys palpable?

Ix
- Urine MC&S (?infection).
- Bloods (U&Es, urea).
- **USS** (to look at anatomy).
- **MCUG** is diagnostic for vesicoureteric reflux.
- Nuclear imaging (DMSA) to identify renal scarring.

DDx
- Other renal disease
- Posterior urethral valves
- Neurogenic bladder

Management

- Recommendations vary depending on grade of disease (see *Fig. 11.3*).

  Mild:
  - **Observation** and advice on identifying features of infection

  Moderate:
  - **Antibiotic prophylaxis** to prevent further damage to the kidneys due to infection

  Severe:
  - **Surgical repair**.
- Spontaneous regression is seen in ~80% of children.

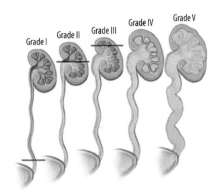

Fig. 11.3: **Grades of vesicoureteric reflux:** from I (mild reflux into a non-dilated ureter) to grade V (severe reflux with dilatation of the renal pelvis).

11.4 Nephrotic syndrome

A **triad** of findings resulting from damage to the **basement membrane** of the glomerulus. It is not a diagnosis in itself; instead, it is a syndrome seen **as a consequence** of other diseases affecting the kidney (see *Table 11.5*).

Table 11.5: Causes of nephrotic syndrome	
Primary causes (renal problem)	**Secondary causes (systemic problem)**
Minimal change disease (most common)	SLE
Primary focal glomerulosclerosis	HSP/other vasculitis
Membranoproliferative glomerulonephritis	Chronic infections (hepatitis, HIV, malaria)
Idiopathic	Diabetes

Pathophysiology

The triad of nephrotic syndrome is **proteinuria, hypoalbuminaemia and oedema**, which can be explained as follows:

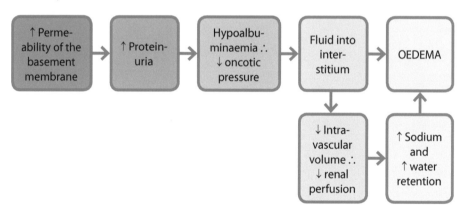

Consequences of nephrotic syndrome:

- **Hypercholesterolaemia** – low serum protein triggers lipid synthesis by the liver.
- **Hypovolaemia** – ↓ intravascular volume due to fluid shifts from hypoalbuminaemia.
- **Thrombosis risk** – hypercoagulable state due to (i) loss of proteins such as antithrombin via the kidneys and (ii) raised haematocrit from hypovolaemia.
- **Infection risk** – especially to encapsulated organisms, because of urinary loss of complement and immunoglobulins (both of which are proteins).

Clinical features

Symptoms

- Oedema (**peripheral** and **periorbital**).
- Poor urine output (→ hypovolaemia).

Signs

- Tachycardia and prolonged cap refill (→ hypovolaemia).
- Infection (loss of complement and immunoglobulins).

Table 11.6: Risk factors for nephrotic syndrome
Male sex
Asian ethnicity
Respiratory tract infections
Family history

Rapid diagnosis – nephrotic syndrome

Nephrotic syndrome consists of:
- Proteinuria >3g/day
- Hypoproteinaemia (albumin <25g/L)
- Oedema
- Hyperlipidaemia

Investigation and diagnosis

Hx
- Acute onset of **abdominal pain**, **malaise**, **lethargy**, with development of **oedema** with **reduced urine output**.
- Ask about diarrhoea and recent infections.

Ex
- Child may be in **hypovolaemic shock (↑ HR and ↓ BP)**.
- **Periorbital oedema** is an early sign ± **scrotal oedema** ± **ascites** ± **peripheral oedema**. A significant minority will be **hypertensive.**
- Pulmonary oedema or pleural effusions with **respiratory distress** may be present.

Ix
- **Urine** (↑ protein, MC&S, sodium concentration).
- **Bloods** (FBC, renal profile, complement, ↓ albumin, ↑ lipids and coagulation).
- **Throat swab** and **ASOT** – for streptococcal detection.
- **Renal biopsy** if steroid resistant/atypical features.

DDx
- Orthostatic proteinuria
- Transient proteinuria
- Nephritic syndrome (if haematuria present)
- Systemic disease with renal involvement

Management

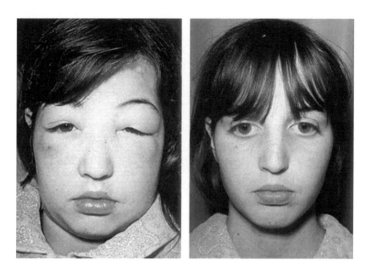

Fig. 11.4: A girl with nephrotic syndrome before and after treatment. Note the dramatic periorbital oedema.

- **High dose prednisolone** (usually 60mg/day) for 4 weeks then a reduced dose for a further 4 weeks; **this treats most cases**.
- **Non-responders** → **biopsy**. Those that **relapse (2/3) need further steroids** and if they continue to relapse (1/3) → immunosuppression.

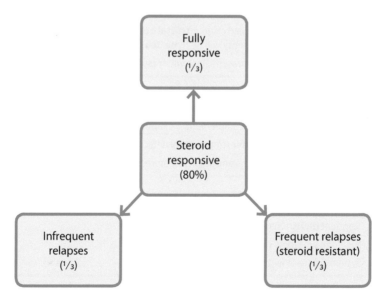

Nephritic syndrome

Nephritic syndrome is a consequence of glomerulonephritis (GN) and is characterized by
1. proteinuria, **2. haematuria**, **3. renal failure** (of variable severity) and **4. hypertension**
(see below).

Pathophysiology

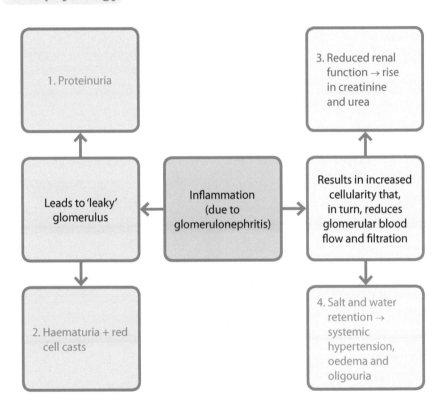

Table 11.7: Main causes of nephritic syndrome	
Post-streptococcal glomerulonephritis (PSGN)	• Most common acute GN, caused by group A strep. • Typically, 2 weeks after throat infection or 6 weeks after skin infection • ASOT positive after most throat infections; check anti-DNAse B titre • Distinguishing feature – C3 is low, C4 is normal
IgA nephropathy	• Commonest cause of chronic GN • Adolescents/young adults • Presentation triggered by URTI → haematuria develops 1–2 days later • Diagnosed on biopsy → IgA deposits in mesangium

(continued)

Table 11.7: (continued)	
Henoch–Schönlein purpura (HSP)	• IgA/IgG/complement complexes deposited in organs causing a vasculitis and subsequent multisystem symptoms • Typically a boy age 3–10 in winter, shortly after an URTI • Abdominal pain, joint pain and characteristic rash on legs (see *Section 15.5.2*)
Glomerular basement membrane disease	• Goodpasture disease (very rare) → antibodies to basement membrane • Alport syndrome → type IV collagen disorder causing abnormal basement membrane; X-linked; associated with sensorineural deafness

Epidemiology

The incidence and prevalence of these conditions are not well understood. Estimates are around 4 per 100 000 children.

Clinical features

Symptoms

- Haematuria (often cola-coloured)
- Oliguria
- Feeling non-specifically unwell
- Symptoms of the aetiology (i.e. preceding infection).

Table 11.8: Risk factors for nephritic syndrome
Male sex (~2:1)
Preceding viral illness/URTI
Preceding throat infection

Signs

- Hypertension
- Oedema (peripheral, peri-orbital or features of pulmonary oedema)
- Signs of the aetiology.

Investigation and diagnosis

> **Hx**
> - **Haematuria/oedema/oligouria**, which may follow a **skin or throat infection**.
> - Urine typically cola–coloured.
> - Chronic causes (such as IgA nephropathy) may be more indolent and present with **intermittent** episodes of **haematuria**.
> - Ask about **hearing** and **family history** of renal disease (→ Alport syndrome).

Ex
- Hypertension and oedema.
- ± features of preceding infection.
- **Neurological exam** – severe hypertension can cause headaches and encephalopathy.

Ix
- **Urine** – ↑ urinary protein. Microscopy (→ **red cell casts**). Send for MC&S.
- **Bloods** (clotting, urea, renal profile, FBC, phosphate, calcium, albumin, ESR).
- **Complement levels** – C3 and C4. In infectious causes, C3 will be low and C4 will be normal. A low C4 indicates a non-infectious cause.
- **ASOT/anti-DNAse titre** & a throat swab (to check for triggering **streptococcal infection**).
- **Renal USS** indicated in all haematuria cases.
- Consider **renal biopsy** if atypical features.

DDx
Broad and must encompass other causes of haematuria:
- UTI
- Trauma
- Renal stones
- Tumours
- Renal vein thrombosis
- Bleeding disorders
- Sickle cell disease
- TB
- Others

Management

Management can be thought of as (a) managing the primary aetiology and (b) managing the features of nephritic syndrome.

Impaired renal function	• **Electrolytes and renal function** need to be closely monitored • In acute renal failure → consider **intensive care** management and **renal filtration/dialysis**
Hypertension	• **Antihypertensives** may be required (typically an ACE inhibitor or calcium channel blocker)
Fluid overload	• **Oral fluid and salt intake should be restricted** • **Consider dialysis** if severe peripheral or pulmonary oedema
Treating the underlying pathology	• **PSGN**: supportive measures only • **IgA nephropathy**: ACE inhibitors or, if persistent or worsening, steroids may be trialled • **HSP**: generally supportive; if significant renal impairment, steroids or immunosuppression

Complex cases (i.e. not post-infectious) should be **discussed with a renal centre**.

Enuresis

Involuntary loss of urine, typically nocturnal, **beyond the developmental age of 5.** It may be **primary** (the child has never achieved continence) or **secondary** (incontinence in a child that has previously been continent for at least 6 months).

Pathophysiology

- Exact pathophysiology unclear and **multifactorial**.
- Enuresis can occur if there is an issue with a) anatomy, b) neurological development and maturity, c) coordination of the somatic and autonomic nervous systems or d) as a combination of the above.

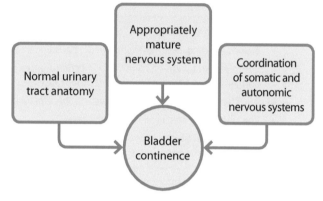

Fig. 11.5: Requirements for bladder continence.

- **Primary: delayed development of the bladder sphincter** (→ likely genetic) is thought to be responsible. Children have smaller bladder capacity and unstable detrusor contractions.
- **Secondary:** should be investigated to find a cause (see *Table 11.9*).

Table 11.9: Causes of enuresis	
Primary causes	**Secondary causes**
Bladder sphincter dysfunction	Diabetes mellitus or insipidus
Neurogenic bladder	Emotional stress
Dysfunctional voiding	UTI or chronic kidney disease (CKD)
Reflux nephropathy or posterior urethral valve causing bladder dysfunction (will be **diurnal**)	Constipation

Epidemiology and risk factors

- **Common.** Seen in up to 15% of 5 year olds and 5% of 10 year olds.
- If both parents affected → 77% chance of children being affected; 44% if 1 parent affected.

Table 11.10: Risk factors for enuresis

Family history	• Genetic component of delayed maturation very likely
Male sex (M:F 2:1)	• Reason for this again unclear
Emotional stress	• In secondary enuresis, thorough history of child's social and emotional wellbeing important
Constipation	• Faecal loading can cause bladder outlet obstruction

Investigation and diagnosis

Hx
- **Characteristics** of enuresis: **daytime, night-time or both** (diurnal)? How often is child passing urine continently? Is the pattern of voiding dysfunctional?
- Ask about **bowel habit**.
- Ask about **stressful life events** and sleeping pattern.
- Ask about **family history** (usually present).
- Ask about **polyuria/polydipsia**, **drinking habits** and caffeine intake (fizzy drinks).

Ex
- **Developmental assessment** – usually normal.
- **Abdominal exam** – for masses (enlarged kidneys, faecal loading). Is the bladder palpable? Is the child hypertensive? (→ suggestive of CKD)
- **Neurological exam** – is there any evidence of pathology causing a neurogenic bladder? Does the spine feel normal? Any evidence of spina bifida? Is anal tone normal?
- **Genitalia exam** – is there congenital anomaly or any evidence of abuse? Has a circumcision damaged the urethra?

Ix
- **Exclude medical cause** – urine dip (to exclude infection).
- **Blood sugar and ketones** – to exclude diabetes mellitus.
- **Imaging** – not for primary nocturnal enuresis but indicated for secondary enuresis and diurnal enuresis (day and night) with **urodynamics ± spinal imaging** if possible neurological cause.

DDx
- DM
- Diabetes insipidus
- UTI
- Sleep disorders

Be confident in your exclusion of emotional, physical or sexual abuse; secondary enuresis may be the only presenting feature.

Management

- If secondary to organic pathology, managing this usually treats the enuresis.
- If no organic pathology, treatment is with **positive reinforcement techniques** (star charts; see *Fig. 11.6*).
- Failing this, **enuresis alarms** may be effective.
- Evening **fluid restriction** is helpful.
- The vast majority of children 'grow out of' enuresis at a rate of 10–15% per year.
- Children with **secondary enuresis** may need **psychological support** if triggered by a stressful life event.
- Medical management is rarely used as 80–90% have recurrence of symptoms once treatment stops.

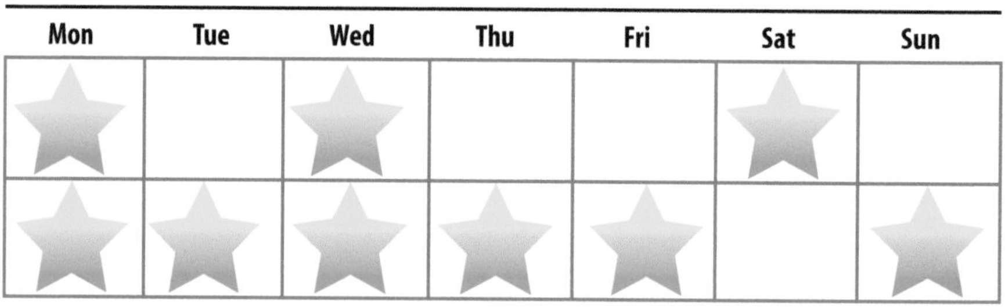

Mon	Tue	Wed	Thu	Fri	Sat	Sun
★		★			★	
★	★	★	★	★		★

Fig. 11.6: Example of a star chart used for positive reinforcement enuresis management. Negativity/chastisement from caregivers gives poor outcomes.

Genital disorders

Almost all genital disorders of childhood are in boys and tend to be related to failure of normal migration of the external genitalia during development *in utero*.

11.7.1 Hypospadia

Pathophysiology

Hypospadia is failure of the urethal folds to close over the urethral groove, so the **urethra opens proximal to the meatus**. The foreskin is hooded dorsally where it has failed to close ventrally. Some more severe hypospadias are associated with a *chordee* (ventral curvature of the penis).

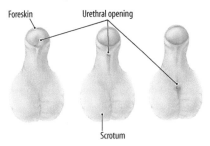

Epidemiology and risk factors

* 1 in 200–500 males.

Table 11.11: Risk factors for hypospadias

Prematurity
Family history

Fig. 11.7: The typical urethral opening in a hypospadias. Note the urethral opening may be anywhere on the shaft or onto the perineum in severe cases.

Investigation and diagnosis

Hx
* Take a detailed **family history** and **urination history**.
* Was the child term or **premature?** If so, what was **birthweight** and exact **gestation?**

Ex
* Obvious hypospadias, large hernias present at birth or cryptorchidism should be identified on the **baby check** prior to discharge after birth.
* **Consent and chaperone for genitalia exam**; with an older child you must enforce that you are a doctor and so you are allowed to examine their genitalia but other people should not be.
* Concurrent cryptorchidism is present in 10% and inguinal hernias are also common.

Ix
* **U&Es** – for severe hypospadias as may cause renal disease.

DDx
* Complex urological tract anomaly

Management

- Surgical correction at around 2 years of age.
- Aim to have urethral opening on meatus so can micturate normally.
- **Must not be circumcised** as this tissue is often needed for surgical correction.

11.7.2 Cryptorchidism

Pathophysiology

Cryptorchidism is the **failure of the testes to follow normal route of descent**. They may be absent, intra-abdominal, or in the inguinal canal.

Testicular descent requires anti-Müllerian hormone (for abdominal descent) and testosterone (→ inguinal canal and scrotum). It is more common in preterm infants as descent through the inguinal canal occurs in the 3rd trimester.

Abdominal (15%)

Inguinal canal (25%)

Prescrotal (65%)

Normal position

Fig. 11.8: The different common positions of an undescended testis. Most (65%) are prescrotal, 25% inguinal and the rest abdominal.

Epidemiology and risk factors

- 1:100 males at 1 year of age.
- 4:100 term males at birth.

Table 11.12: Risk factors for cryptorchidism

Prematurity
Family history

Investigation and diagnosis

Hx
- Take a detailed **family history** and **urination history**.
- Do the **testes/scrotum change when the child is being bathed**? This may be the case in retractile rather than undescended testes, or in an inguinal hernia.
- Was the child term or **premature?** If so, what was **birthweight** and exact **gestation**?

Ex
- An empty scrotum unilaterally or bilaterally should be noted at newborn baby check.
- **Consent and chaperone for genitalia exam**; with an older child you must enforce that you are a doctor and so you are allowed to examine their genitalia but other people should not be.

Ix
- **USS** – to identify where the testes are, rule out hernias.

> **DDx**
> - Retractile testes
> - Ectopic testes
> - Absent testes

Management

- Surgical correction (**orchidopexy**) at 1 year of age. Fertility deteriorates the later the corrective surgery is performed.
- Education and surveillance for **malignancy**, 5 × higher rate of testicular cancer in early adulthood (20–30 years) in this group.
- Counselling on **infertility risk** in adulthood.

Rapid diagnosis – retractile testes

An excessive cremasteric reflex, causing the testes to retract **into the inguinal canal**. They will spontaneously descend back into the scrotum in the warm, or can be manipulated back. They are **normal and common,** but require follow-up until puberty to ensure they do not become 'ascending' (→ fixed outside of the scrotum i.e. secondary cryptorchidism – **rare**).

Chapter 12

Neurological disorders

Meningitis

Meningitis is a serious infection and, although rare, is the leading cause of death in early childhood.

Pathophysiology

Inflammation of the arachnoid mater, pia mater and CSF, which is either viral (common) or bacterial (rarer).

- Viral:
  - Enteroviruses (such as Coxsackie virus and Echovirus) – most common; herpes simplex virus (HSV); varicella zoster virus (VZV); HIV.
- Bacterial:
  - Neonates: *Streptococcus agalactiae; Haemophilus influenzae* Type B (HIB)
  - Childhood: *Neisseria meningitidis* (most common); *Streptococcus pneumoniae*

Bacteria and viruses tend to spread to the meninges via the haematogenous route, where they cause an inflammatory reaction.

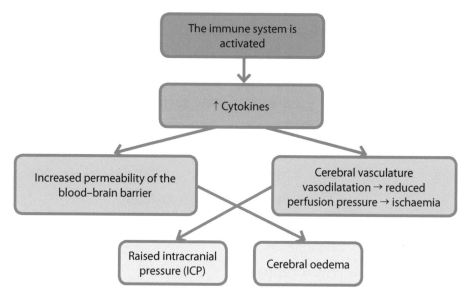

 Children with a *N. meningitidis* infection can develop **meningococcal septicaemia** as the bacteria release an **endotoxin** that, through a cascade, can result in:
- Increased vascular permeability → may lead to hypovolaemia
- Coagulopathy → petechiae and purpura
- Myocardial dysfunction
- Metabolic disturbance – acidosis, $\downarrow K^+$, $\downarrow Ca^{2+}$, $\downarrow Mg^{2+}$

Epidemiology and risk factors

Table 12.1: Risk factors for meningitis

Maternal infection	Splenectomy
Premature rupture of membranes (PROM)	Not immunized
Low birthweight	CSF shunt
Prematurity	Immunocompromised

Clinical features

Viral meningitis is less significant than bacterial disease and usually managed conservatively; however, **all cases must be managed as <u>bacterial</u> meningitis <u>until proven otherwise</u>**.

Table 12.2: Features of meningitis in infants and children

	Symptoms	Signs
Meningeal irritation	Neck stiffness Photophobia	Brudzinski sign Kernig sign Seizures
Raised ICP + cerebral oedema	Altered consciousness Nausea/vomiting	↓GCS Bulging of fontanelles (<2 y/o) Papilloedema (Focal neurology)
Cytokine release	Rigors Headache	Fever
Meningococcal septicaemia: • ↑ vascular permeability • Coagulopathy	Hypovolaemia Non-blanching rash	↓BP, ↑HR Petechiae and purpura

Rapid diagnosis – meningitis in the neonate

Features in neonates are less characteristic of meningitis and it should therefore be considered in any unwell neonate. In general, the neonate is irritable, listless, poorly feeding and looks unwell.

OSCE tips 1: Brudzinski and Kernig signs (see *Fig. 12.1*)

Brudzinski
Child is supine. Passively flex their neck, and they have a <u>reflex flexion</u> of their hips.

Kernig
Patient supine. Passively flex hip and knee to 90°. Then passively straighten the knee – this will produce <u>pain along the spine</u>.

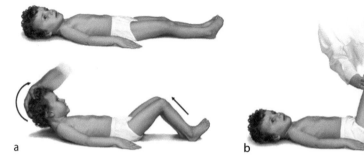

Fig. 12.1: (a) Brudzinski and (b) Kernig signs.

Investigation and diagnosis

Hx
- An unwell, febrile child with features of meningeal irritation and raised ICP.
- The classic symptoms are fever, headache, photophobia and neck stiffness.
- Ask about a non-blanching rash.

Ex
- Unwell and febrile. Look for signs of shock.
- Look for petechiae.
- Examine for Brudzinski and Kernig signs.
- Examine for features of ↑ ICP (↓ GCS, sluggish pupils, focal neurology, papilloedema).

Ix
- Blood cultures, FBC, CRP, renal profile.
- Lumbar puncture with CSF analysis is gold standard, **but is contraindicated if there are features of raised ICP.**
  - Note that CSF glucose level is **relative** to plasma glucose level, a sample of which should be taken and sent to the lab at the same time as the CSF.

	Appearance	White cells	Protein content	Glucose content
Bacterial	Turbid	Neutrophils	↑↑↑	↓↓↓
Viral	Clear	Lymphocytes	–/ ↑	–/ ↓

DDx
- Any cause of sepsis
- Intracranial abscess
- Encephalitis
- Intracranial tumours
- Hydrocephalus

Management

Do not delay starting empirical antibiotics whilst awaiting diagnostic tests:
- ABCDE with resuscitation as needed
- IV antibiotics
- IV corticosteroids (if >3 months of age)

OSCE tips 2: Complications of meningitis

'SAD REP is Deaf':

Sepsis/Shock/SIADH, **A**taxia/Abscess, **D**IC, **R**etardation, **E**pilepsy, **P**aralysis, **Deaf**ness

Pathophysiology

A seizure that is associated with **fever**, and is **unrelated to other pathology** (such as neurological infection and sepsis). The majority of children have a viral URTI, although any febrile condition can lead to a febrile convulsion.

 It is important to recognize that more sinister pathology can present as a seizure; consequently, a careful history and examination are paramount for safe decision-making.

Epidemiology and risk factors

Between 1 and 5 years of age, ~1 in 20 children will suffer a febrile convulsion. They recur in 1/3 of children but **should not happen >5 y/o**. Family history (maternal > paternal) is the most important risk factor.

Diagnosis and investigation

Hx
- A preceding febrile illness **must** be evident.
- Generalized tonic-clonic seizure, lasting ~5 mins (and <15 mins).
- **No features** of meningitis, encephalitis or sepsis.
- Full recovery <1 hr.

Ex
- Febrile. Other observations near normal. GCS 15 within 1 hr.
- Systemically well with **no features** of meningitis, encephalitis or sepsis – petechial rash, vomiting, headache, neck stiffness, bulging fontanelle.
- No focal neurology.

Ix
- A clinical diagnosis.
- Where there is doubt –
  - Bloods
  - MSU
  - ± LP (?infective changes).

DDx
- Febrile – meningitis, encephalitis, sepsis, UTI
- Afebrile – epilepsy, ↓ glucose, electrolyte disturbance, brain injury (consider NAHI), breath-holding spells, reflex anoxic seizure

Management [adapted from NICE CKS]

- Febrile convulsions can be managed at home; where there is doubt, admit for observation ± investigation.
- Advice on **parental management** of seizure (*OSCE tips 3*).
- Manage fever (does not prevent recurrence, however).

OSCE tips 3: Initial management of seizures

- Parents: protect child, do not restrain (→ fracture), nothing in mouth, recovery position after seizure, 999 if >5 mins.
- Doctor: as for parents, plus medical management if seizure >5 mins → rectal diazepam or oral midazolam (Buccolam).

Epilepsy is a common disease that can have profound consequences for the child. In the broadest terms, it is **an enduring predisposition to generating unprovoked seizures**. The International League Against Epilepsy (ILAE) defined the specific diagnostic criteria in 2014 as **any** of the following:

- ≥2 unprovoked seizures occurring >24 hours apart
- 1 unprovoked seizure and a probability of further seizures after 2 unprovoked seizures, occurring over the next 10 years
- Diagnosis of an epilepsy syndrome (i.e. Lennox–Gastaut, Dravet, infantile spasms)

Pathophysiology

An ↑ activation or ↓ inhibition of neurones can lead to an imbalance being created, so causing an overall net excitation → paroxysmal discharge. The brain region affected dictates the symptoms associated with the seizure (see *Table 12.3*):

Table 12.3: Brain regions affected by epilepsy

Lobe	Area affected	Features
Frontal	Motor cortex	Movement impairment
	Frontal cortex	Emotional/cognitive change
Temporal	Auditory cortex	Ringing or hissing/hearing music
	Wernicke's area	Dysphasia
	Olfactory area	Unusual taste or smell
	Superior temporal gyrus	Automatisms, lip smacking, chewing
Parietal	Sensory cortex	Sensory disturbance
Occipital	Visual cortex	Flashes, scotoma or blurring/formed visual hallucinations
Limbic	Amygdala, thalamus and hypothalamus	Autonomic dysfunction

Seizures may be either 'focal' (originating in a single region of the brain, on one side only) or 'generalized' (where a large region of both hemispheres is involved), and focal can progress to generalized during the seizure. Consciousness **may be** affected in focal seizures, but is **always** affected during generalized seizures.

The classification can be summarized as shown in *Fig. 12.2* (adapted from ILAE 2017).

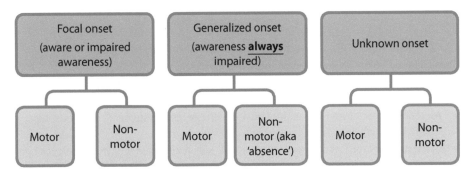

Fig. 12.2: Types of epilepsy.

Epidemiology and risk factors

Approximately 7 in 1000 children are affected.

Risk factors:
- Learning disability
- First-degree relative affected

There are many aetiologies which may cause epilepsy, which include:

• Idiopathic
• Genetic syndromes such as tuberous sclerosis, Rett syndrome and Prader–Willi syndrome
• Metabolic disease
• Mitochondrial disease
• Intracranial infection
• Post-traumatic
• Electrolyte disturbance (high glucose, low Ca^{2+}, low Mg^{2+}, high or low Na^+)

Rapid diagnosis – common (1 & 2) and rare (3–5) epilepsy syndromes

1. Childhood absence epilepsy: ~10% of childhood epilepsies. Frequent absence seizures with onset ~6 years of age.
2. Juvenile myoclonic epilepsy: ~5% of childhood epilepsies. Onset in adolescence and characterized by myoclonic, tonic-clonic and absence seizures. Relative affected in 50% of patients.
3. Dravet syndrome: severe myoclonic epilepsy, which is aggressive and resistant to anti-epileptic drugs (AEDs).
4. Lennox–Gastaut syndrome: multiple seizure types with cognitive impairment.
5. Infantile spasms (West syndrome): 3–9 months of age and characterized by brief myoclonic spasms after waking.

Clinical features

Symptoms and signs

These depend on the seizure type, as shown in *Fig. 12.2*:

- **Focal motor**: up to a few minutes' duration. Characterized by automatisms, tonic/clonic/atonic/myoclonic, affecting **specific region** of body.
- **Focal non-motor**: altered sensation, unusual smell/taste, visual disturbance or hallucinations, autonomic disturbance.
- **Generalized motor**: loss of awareness, associated with motor symptoms (tonic-clonic/tonic/clonic/atonic/myoclonic).
  - The most common type is tonic-clonic. These typically last for 1–3 minutes and are characterized by an initial rigid phase (in which the child falls to the floor), **in which the child may bite their tongue**. This is followed by a rhythmic, jerking phase, during which the child **may lose control of the bladder and bowels**.
  - Afterwards, there is a '**post-ictal**' **phase** – normally lasting from 5–30 minutes, during which the child is drowsy and confused.
- **Generalized (absence) non-motor ('petit mal')**: a very **brief** period (<10s) during which the child stops what they're doing, becomes **unaware**, and **stares** into the distance. It self-terminates and the child resumes what they were doing, with **no post-ictal phase**. This may be confused with day-dreaming.

OSCE tips 4: Definitions of motor terms

- Tonic: stiffness in the limbs
- Clonic: sustained rhythmical jerking of the limbs
- Tonic-clonic ('grand mal'): initial stiffening, followed by jerking
- Atonic: sudden loss of muscle tone, so the child falls to the floor
- Myoclonic: a brief muscle jerk
- Automatisms: repetitive, purposeless actions (such as making sounds, picking at clothes, lip smacking, chewing).

Investigation and diagnosis

Hx
- Ask carefully about events **before, during and after** the episode:
  - Warnings? Triggers? How has the child been recently?
  - Was the child aware or unaware? What movements occurred? Tongue biting or incontinence? How long did it last?
  - Confused? Sleepy? How long until they were back to normal?
- Any family history of epilepsy?

Ex
- Vital signs? Normal growth?
- Any features of chromosomal abnormality or other congenital disease?
- Skin changes (i.e. suggesting tuberous sclerosis)?
- Raised ICP? Head injury?
- Assess peripheral neurology, cerebellum and cranial nerves.

Ix
- Consider bloods to look at electrolytes
- ECG
- EEG (which includes photic stimulation and hyperventilation) – used only to **support** an epilepsy diagnosis, not exclude it. Typically done after the 2nd seizure in children. If not useful, perform a sleep EEG.
- MRI – especially useful if focal seizures ($\rightarrow$?structural brain abnormality) or if <2 years old.

Management

An anti-epileptic drug (AED) is started once the diagnosis is confirmed.

Table 12.4: First-line treatment using AEDs	
Focal seizures	Carbamazepine or lamotrigine
Generalized tonic-clonic seizures	Sodium valproate or lamotrigine
Generalized non-motor (absence)	Ethosuximide or sodium valproate
Myoclonic	Sodium valproate (or levetiracetam if unsuitable)
Tonic or atonic	Sodium valproate (or lamotrigine if unsuitable)

Clinical pharmacology – sodium valproate

Valproate should not be prescribed to female children or adolescents due to its teratogenic effects. Other side-effects can be remembered using the acronym 'VALPROATE' – **V**alproate, **A**taxia, **L**iver failure, **P**ancreatitis, **R**eversible hair loss, **O**edema, **A**ppetite increased, **T**eratogenic/thrombocytopenia, **E**nzyme (CYP450) inhibitor.

Conditions commonly reported as seizures

Breath-holding spells

Pathophysiology

Breath-holding spells (BHS) are a characteristic sequence of events of uncertain aetiology, divided into **cyanotic** and **pallid** types, as outlined below. Onset is 6–18 months of age, with **spontaneous resolution** occurring between 4 and 8 years old.

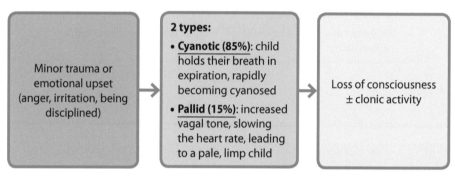

Minor trauma or emotional upset (anger, irritation, being disciplined)

→

2 types:
- **Cyanotic (85%)**: child holds their breath in expiration, rapidly becoming cyanosed
- **Pallid (15%)**: increased vagal tone, slowing the heart rate, leading to a pale, limp child

→

Loss of consciousness ± clonic activity

Epidemiology and risk factors

- 5% of children
- Associated with iron-deficiency anaemia
- ~1/3 have a positive family history.

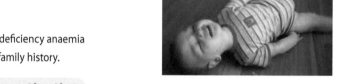

Fig. 12.3: Infant during BHS.

Diagnosis and investigation

Hx
- **A typical sequence** of events following minor injury/upset, leading to unconsciousness.
- Quick resolution of symptoms (no post-ictal phase).

Ex
- During the episode – cyanosis/pallor and limpness.

Ix
- Bloods – ?iron deficiency
- ECG – ?long QT syndrome
- EEG – normal in BHS

DDx
- Seizure
- Arrhythmia
- Long QT syndrome
- Tics
- Reflux

Management

- Make the area safe to avoid injury and do not restrain.
- Blowing on the child's face has been reported to terminate the episode in some.
- Reinforce rules and avoid tantrums.
- Treat anaemia if present.
- Reassurance for the parents is important: BHS are distressing.

12.4.2 Tics

Pathophysiology

Tics are purposeless sudden, rapid, recurrent, non-rhythmic motor movements or vocalizations, the pathophysiology of which is poorly understood, but likely multifactorial. They may be (i) **motor**, **vocal**, **sensory** or **cognitive**, and (ii) **simple** or **complex**.

Table 12.5: Types of tic				
	Motor	**Vocal**	**Sensory**	**Cognitive**
Simple	Blinking, shrugging	Coughing, sniffing	Unpleasant sensations relieved by execution of the tic	Repetitive thoughts
Complex	Mimicking, elaborate movements	Repeating others or oneself, obscene phrases		

Tic disorders have a **high association with attention deficit hyperactivity disorder (ADHD), obsessive–compulsive disorder (OCD) and learning difficulties**. Additionally, it is important to recognize that tics may be secondary to another underlying diagnosis (see DDx box, below).

Epidemiology and risk factors

Tic disorders may occur in <20% of children and **family history increases risk by 10–100x**. Onset is typically ~5–6 y/o.

Diagnosis and investigation

Hx
- Triggers? Functional impact?
- Features of a secondary cause?
- Features of an associated condition?

Ex
- **Observation** of the child (clinic/video).
- Thorough neurological assessment, which **should be normal**.

> **Ix** Only required where the history/examination is not typical, consider:
> - TFTs and streptococcal throat swab
> - MRI of brain
> - EEG

DDx

Drugs	Neurodegenerative	Infective	Other
• Stimulants • Anti-convulsants • Antihistamines	• Huntington disease • Wilson disease	• Encephalitis • Variant Creutzfeldt–Jakob disease (vCJD) • Post-streptococcal (PANDAS or Sydenham chorea)	• Hyper-thyroidism • Epilepsy

Management

- Treat secondary causes if present.
- Habit reversal therapy.
- Pharmacologically with clonidine and antipsychotic medications (i.e. risperidone, haloperidol, olanzapine).

Rapid diagnosis – Tourette syndrome

Diagnostic criteria (clinical):
- ≥2 motor and ≥1 vocal tic
- Present for ≥12 months
- Onset <18 years old
- Tics not caused by other conditions (e.g. Huntington's) or medications

12.4.3 Self-gratification

Pathophysiology

A **normal behaviour** seen in childhood that can be mistaken for epilepsy, dystonias or dyskinesias, particularly in young infants. Recognition is therefore important to reduce unnecessary investigation.

Epidemiology and risk factors

Two peaks in childhood – between **3 months and 3 years** and again in adolescence. It is reported in ~90% of males and 50% of females.

Diagnosis and investigation

Hx Repetitive and **stereotyped** episodes, with characteristic features:

- Dystonic posturing
- Child appears distracted
- Clinical features
- Grunting
- Normal GCS
- Facial flushing & sweating

Ix
- Not required.
- Home recording of the event can prevent unnecessary investigation.

DDx
- Seizures
- Dystonia
- Dyskinesia

Management

- Counselling and education of the parents (→ this is a normal behaviour).
- Distraction can help redirect the child's attention.
- The behaviour will usually self-terminate.

OSCE tips 5: Key neurological terminology

An appreciation of the variety of neurological symptoms is important; these are best understood and remembered through clinical observation.

Term	Definition
Ataxia	Unsteady, broad-based gait
Athetosis	Writhing, slow movements
Chorea	Unpredictable, irregular, non-rhythmic movements
Dyskinesia	A broad term for any involuntary, abnormal movement
Dystonia	Repetitive twisting movement and postures, often sustained
Myoclonus	Brief, sudden involuntary movements
Torticollis	A dystonia specifically affecting the neck
Tremor	Rhythmic oscillation of a body part

12.4.4 Night terrors

A common condition within the group of disorders termed 'parasomnias', the pathophysiology of which is not well understood. It is commonly associated with sleepwalking and characterized by **sudden arousal from sleep** during the non-rapid eye movement phase.

Epidemiology and risk factors

- Estimated prevalence of 1–6% (DSM-IV), with a **peak prevalence at 3.5 years of age**.
- Risk is increased in those with an affected first-degree relative.

Diagnosis and investigation

Hx
- Sudden shouting/screaming and **sympathetic overdrive** (↑HR, ↑RR, sweating).
- The child is initially unresponsive and confused.
- Enuresis may be present.
- No recall of events.

Ix
- Sleep diary.
- **Consider EEG if features of nocturnal seizures.**

DDx
- Epilepsy
- Post-traumatic stress disorder
- Panic attacks
- Neuropsychiatric disorders
- Child abuse

Management

- Often not required, with spontaneous resolution before their teenage years common.
- **Conservative measures** to prevent the child from harming themselves during the episode may be needed.

Rapid diagnosis – parasomnias

Night terrors are part of a group of conditions termed 'parasomnias': unwanted events that occur whilst falling asleep, sleeping or waking up.

Sleepwalking is seen in ~5% of children and is most prevalent between 3 and 7 years of age. The child tends to walk around the home with their eyes open, although they are unresponsive during the episode. An episode usually lasts around 10 minutes. The child should be gently ushered back to bed, where they will generally fall back asleep. Conservative measures to ensure safety are essential:

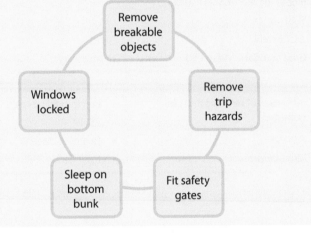

12.4.5 Psychogenic non-epileptic seizures

Pathophysiology

Psychogenic non-epileptic seizures (PNES) may mimic, and so be misdiagnosed as, epileptic seizures. Instead, PNES is a **psychiatric disorder**.

Epidemiology and risk factors

Approximately 1 in 5 referrals for non-medication-responsive epilepsy are due to PNES, with around 80% of PNES patients having initially been treated for epilepsy. There is an increased incidence in those with mental health and personality disorders.

Diagnosis and investigation

Hx
- Stress and emotional upset are common antecedents.
- Stressors that *reliably* cause a seizure are suggestive of PNES.
- More likely to occur in front of an audience.
- **Rarely** occur during sleep.

Ex
- **Gradual**, rather than sudden, onset.
- Eyes closed.
- Shaking head from **side to side**.
- **Asynchronous, flailing** limbs.
- Arching of the back.
- **Recall** of the event.

Ix
- Bloods inc. electrolytes and BM
- ECG
- ± CT or MRI
- **Gold standard**: **video EEG** → **normal** electrical activity

DDx
- **All causes of seizures must be excluded**
- Syncope
- Night terrors
- Breath-holding spells
- ADHD
- Factitious disorder
- Malingering

Management

- *A sensitive discussion about the diagnosis is important to good outcomes*: the patient is not 'faking' the episodes.
- AEDs are of no value.
- Treatment of co-morbid mental health conditions, if present.
- Cognitive behavioural therapy may be of value.

Rapid diagnosis – factitious disorders vs. malingering

- **Factitious disorder**: physical or mental health symptoms are **consciously falsified**, with the **subconscious aim** of being 'looked after', but no other discernable benefit. This often leads to unnecessary diagnostic procedures, which may be invasive, that the patient often accepts with equanimity.
- **Malingering**: symptoms are **consciously** falsified, but they have a clear, **conscious** motivation for doing so (e.g. financial gain or avoiding responsibilities).

Headaches

Headaches are a common presenting symptom that, whilst **often benign** in origin, may be due to a sinister pathology – a comprehensive history and examination are therefore essential in the correct diagnosis and work-up of these children.

Pathophysiology

Headaches can be classified as **primary** (→ attributable to a headache disorder) or **secondary** (→ due to another underlying disease). By considering the anatomical structures that can cause headache, one can determine the aetiologies:

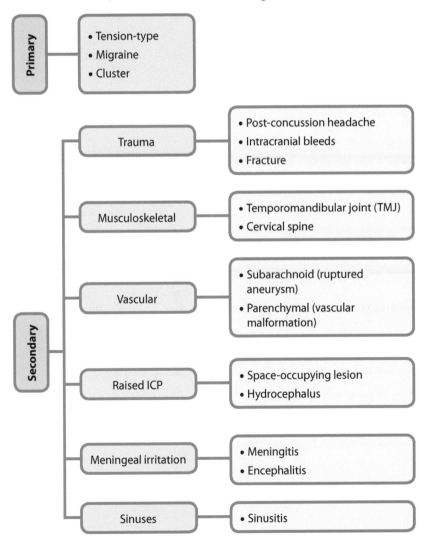

Primary
- Tension-type
- Migraine
- Cluster

Secondary

Trauma
- Post-concussion headache
- Intracranial bleeds
- Fracture

Musculoskeletal
- Temporomandibular joint (TMJ)
- Cervical spine

Vascular
- Subarachnoid (ruptured aneurysm)
- Parenchymal (vascular malformation)

Raised ICP
- Space-occupying lesion
- Hydrocephalus

Meningeal irritation
- Meningitis
- Encephalitis

Sinuses
- Sinusitis

Clinical features

Diagnosis	Features of headache	Possible associated symptoms
Tension	Bilateral or posterior; tight; unaffected by routine activity	Nil
Migraine	Unilateral or bilateral; pulsating; severe	Nausea/vomiting; photophobia; phonophobia; ± 'aura' ($\rightarrow$ visual/sensory/speech disturbance)
Cluster	Unilateral, around the eye; stabbing/throbbing/burning; severe	Characteristically, ipsilateral red eye, epiphora, nasal congestion and sweating
Sinusitis	Frontal	Facial tenderness; nasal congestion; sore ear; cough; fever
Meningitis	Generalized	Unwell; fever; stiff neck; rash; focal neurology
Encephalitis	Generalized	Fever; altered mental status (drowsy/confused); ± seizures; ± $\downarrow$GCS
Space-occupying lesion	Localized or generalized; slowly worsening; worse in the mornings; worse with Valsalva manoeuvre	Vomiting; focal neurology (~90%); altered personality
Haemorrhage	Sudden onset; often follows trauma	$\downarrow$GCS; focal neurology; seizures
TMJ	Unilateral or bilateral; worse with jaw movement	$\downarrow$ mandibular movement

Epidemiology and risk factors

Very common $\rightarrow$ ~50% <10 y/o and 75% <15 y/o.

Investigation and diagnosis

Hx
- Position and characteristics
- Onset (?Trauma ?Sudden)
- Aggravating factors ($\rightarrow$ Valsalva and position)
- Change over time (? $\uparrow$ in frequency)
- Associated symptoms:
  - Neurology – neck stiffness, focal neurology, visual disturbance, seizures, altered consciousness, behavioural changes
  - ENT – coryzal symptoms, sore ears/eyes/throat
  - GI – nausea and vomiting
  - Dermatology – rash
  - Systemic – fevers

Ex
- Vital signs including GCS
- Skin – rashes
- ENT assessment
- Eyes – pupils and fundoscopy ($\rightarrow$?papilloedema)
- Neck – Kernig and Brudzinski signs; C-spine range of motion
- Neurology:
  - Cranial nerves
  - Peripheral neurology – tone, power, reflexes, coordination, sensation
  - Cerebellum $\rightarrow$ DANISH
  - Gait

Ix
- Bloods – ? $\uparrow$inflammatory markers
- Lumbar puncture (if suspected intracranial infection or idiopathic intracranial hypertension)
- CT head $\pm$ MRI brain (if features of infection, haemorrhage, space-occupying lesion or raised intracranial pressure)

Management

- Headache diary
- Treat secondary headaches as you would the underlying diagnosis
- Treat primary headaches as follows [adapted from NICE 2012, CG150 (for children >12 y/o)]:

Tension-type	Migraine	Cluster
• Paracetamol or NSAID	• Acute: oral triptan + NSAID or paracetamol ± anti-emetic • Prophylaxis: topiramate or propranolol	• Acute: oxygen + SC/IM triptan (oral not useful acutely) • Paracetamol/NSAIDs/opioids not useful • Prophylaxis: verapamil 1st line

12.6 Hydrocephalus

Hydrocephalus is a **rise in CSF volume** within the central nervous system → raised ICP.

Pathophysiology

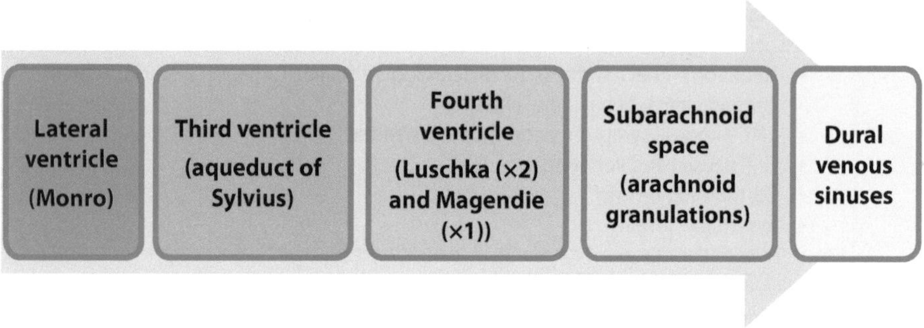

| Lateral ventricle (Monro) | Third ventricle (aqueduct of Sylvius) | Fourth ventricle (Luschka (×2) and Magendie (×1)) | Subarachnoid space (arachnoid granulations) | Dural venous sinuses |

Fig. 12.4: Flow of CSF through the ventricles – the foramina connecting each of them are in parentheses.

Table 12.6: Types of hydrocephalus – non-communicating vs. communicating

Type	Non-communicating	Communicating
Pathophysiology	There is an **obstruction to the flow** of CSF through the ventricular system (or between the 4th ventricle and the subarachnoid space)	↓ **drainage** of CSF from the subarachnoid space (through the arachnoid granulations) or, rarely, ↑ **production** of CSF
Aetiologies	Arnold–Chiari malformation; Dandy–Walker malformation; space-occupying lesions (tumour, abscess, haematoma, cysts); intraventricular haemorrhage; stenosis of aqueduct	Post-meningitis; choroid plexus papilloma; increased venous sinus pressure (e.g. achondroplasia or venous thrombosis)

Epidemiology and risk factors

~3–5 per 1000 live births. Most patients present <2 y/o.

Table 12.7: Risk factors for hydrocephalus

Congenital abnormalities
Intraventricular haemorrhage

Clinical features

Symptoms

- In infants: irritability, poor feeding, vomiting.
- In children: those of raised ICP – headaches/vomiting worse in the morning ± reduced GCS; blurred/double vision; difficulty walking.

Signs

- In infants: macrocephaly, bulging fontanelle, 'setting-sun' sign (*Fig. 12.5*) – eyes downward with upper lid retracted, upper motor neurone (UMN) signs – hypertonia and spasticity (lower limb > upper limb).
- In children:
  - UMN signs: spasticity and hypertonia → unsteady on feet
  - Eyes: papilloedema; failure of upward gaze; CN VI palsy (due to long intracranial course)
  - Macewen sign: percussion of the head results in a 'cracked pot' sound

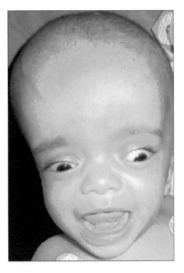

Fig. 12.5: The 'setting-sun' sign plus macrocephaly, symptomatic of hydrocephalus.

Investigation and diagnosis

Hx	• An irritable child with features of raised intracranial pressure, UMN symptoms and ocular symptoms.

Ex	• General inspection may reveal an unwell child with an enlarged head. • Assess their GCS and examine for peripheral neurology (UMN signs). • Look in the eyes of older children.

Ix	• Imaging: USS through the infant's fontanelles/CT brain in older children. • An MRI is useful to look for the Arnold–Chiari malformation or small tumours.

DDx	• Intracranial tumour • Intracranial haemorrhage • Meningitis • Epilepsy • Migraine

Management

 Hydrocephalus with a raised ICP is a surgical emergency.
Definitive treatment is surgical decompression via placement of a **ventricular shunt**. The most common definitive measure is a ventriculoperitoneal (VP) shunt (*Fig. 12.6*) or, as a temporizing measure, an extraventricular drain.

Rapid diagnosis

- **Arnold–Chiari malformation**: a spectrum of **hindbrain anomalies** which ultimately results in **cerebellar herniation** through the foramen magnum → disruption of CSF drainage.
  - Type I: >5mm herniation of the cerebellar tonsils through the foramen magnum.
  - Type II: brainstem, 4th ventricle and cerebellar vermian displacement through the foramen magnum; more severe and typically seen with a myelomeningocele.

- **Dandy–Walker malformation**: a rare malformation which broadly includes:
  - Large 4th ventricular cyst
  - An enlarged, bossed posterior cranial fossa
  - Absence/hypoplasia of the cerebellar vermis.

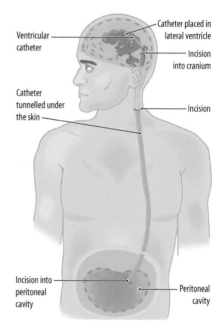

Ventricular catheter

Catheter placed in lateral ventricle

Incision into cranium

Catheter tunnelled under the skin

Incision

Incision into peritoneal cavity

Peritoneal cavity

Fig. 12.6: A VP shunt. They may become blocked (↑ICP), infected (≤6 months after placement) or cause abdominal complications.

12.7 Neurocutaneous disorders

These are a group of conditions that largely affect tissues of **ectodermal origin** (the nervous system and skin), although other tissues may be involved. The most important conditions to be aware of are neurofibromatosis (NF) and tuberous sclerosis.

12.7.1 Neurofibromatosis

Pathophysiology

An **autosomal dominant** genetic disorder categorized into two types: NF1 (mutation on chromosome 17q → ↓ neurofibromin) and NF2 (chromosome 22q → ↓ merlin). These genes serve as **tumour suppressors**, and aberrations therefore predispose to the **development of tumours within the nervous system** – these are **usually benign**, but may be malignant.

NF1 is a multisystem disorder, whereas NF2 mainly affects the central nervous system.

Epidemiology and risk factors

Incidence: NF1 ~1:4000 and NF2 ~1:50 000. The main risk factor is a **family history** of NF.

Clinical features

Note that NF is a heterogenous condition and clinical features vary widely (see *Fig. 12.7*)

Neurological
- Learning disability
- Motor delay
- Epilepsy
- Palpable peripheral nerve plexiform neurofibromas

Cutaneous
- Cutaneous neurofibromas
- Café au lait spots
- Axillary or inguinal freckling

NF1

Musculoskeletal
- Scoliosis
- Anterolateral tibial bowing
- Radial and ulnar bowing

Others
- CV: congenital heart disease
- GI: abdo pain, constipation, bleeding
- Endocrine: phaeochromocytoma

Ocular
- Optic nerve glioma (visual field defect)
- Lisch nodules (iris hamartoma)

Fig. 12.7: Features of NF1.

NF2 is characterized by the presence of **bilateral vestibular schwannomas** (→ tinnitus, hearing loss and poor balance) ± other central nervous system tumours (neurofibroma, meningioma, glioma). Cutaneous manifestations are less prominent.

Investigation and diagnosis

Ix
- A clinical diagnosis (see below).
- Slit lamp to look for Lisch nodules.
- Hearing tests if vestibulocochlear nerve involved.
- Consider X-ray (long bones) and MRI brain.

DDx
- McCune–Albright syndrome
- Legius syndrome

Rapid diagnosis – NF1	Rapid diagnosis – NF2

Require ≥2 of:
• >5 café au lait spots (*Fig. 12.8a*)
• Axillary/inguinal freckling (*Fig. 12.8b*)
• ≥2 neurofibromas (or 1 plexiform neurofibroma) (*Fig. 12.8c*)
• Optic nerve glioma
• ≥2 Lisch nodules (*Fig. 12.8d*)
• Long bone abnormalities (as described above)
• 1st-degree relative with NF1
	Require ≥1 of:
	• Bilateral vestibulocochlear nerve masses (vestibular schwannomas)
	• Unilateral vestibulocochlear nerve masses and 1st-degree relative with NF2
	• 1st-degree relative with NF2 + ≥2 of:
	  • Meningioma
	  • Glioma
	  • Schwannoma
	  • Juvenile cataract

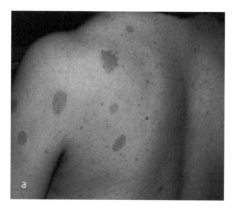
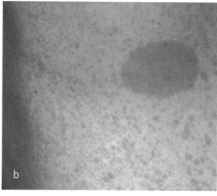

Fig. 12.8: Features of NF1: (a) Café au lait spots; (b) axillary freckling.

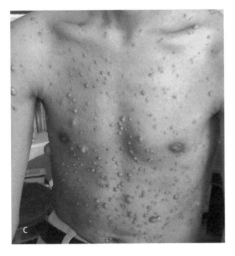
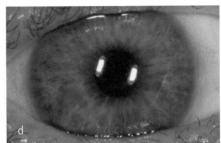

Fig. 12.8: Features of NF1 (*continued*): (c) neurofibromas; (d) Lisch nodules.

Management

- There is no curative treatment; management is therefore based on identifying and treating complications as they arise.
- Annual clinical examination and eye tests.
- Genetic counselling of the older child.
- Orthopaedic input for long bone deformities or scoliosis.
- Neurofibromas that are causing compressive pathology need urgent surgical attention, although recurrence is common.
- Malignant tumours require immediate attention.

Rapid diagnosis – other neurocutaneous disorders

- **Sturge–Weber syndrome:** angiomas affecting the skin and meninges. Characterized by the presence of a **facial port-wine stain**. Seizures and cognitive deficit are common.
- **von Hippel–Lindau: 'HIPPEL'** – **H**aemangioblastoma; **I**ncreased RCC (~60%); **P**haeochromocytoma; **P**ancreatic lesions; **E**ye dysfunction; **L**iver, renal and pancreatic cysts.

12.7.2 Tuberous sclerosis

Tuberous sclerosis is an **autosomal dominant** disease characterized by **multisystem hamartomas** (→ commonly in the brain, skin and kidneys), affecting ~1 in 6000 children.

Pathophysiology

The *TSC1* gene (→ hamartin) or *TSC2* gene (→ tuberin) may be affected; together, they form a tumour suppressor gene. Mutations therefore predispose to **unregulated cell growth**.

Diagnosis and investigation

<u>**Often presents as seizures**</u> (due to cortical tubers), but clinical manifestations vary. The major multisystem manifestations of tuberous sclerosis are shown in *Fig. 12.9*.

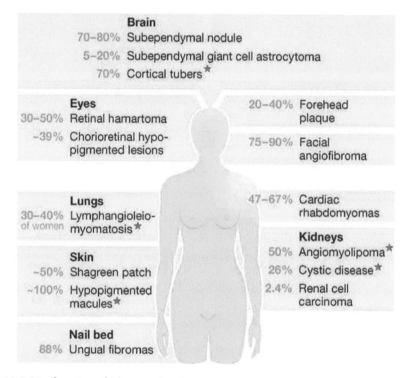

Brain
70–80% Subependymal nodule
5–20% Subependymal giant cell astrocytoma
70% Cortical tubers*

Eyes
30–50% Retinal hamartoma
~39% Chorioretinal hypo-pigmented lesions

20–40% Forehead plaque
75–90% Facial angiofibroma

Lungs
30–40% Lymphangioleio-
of women myomatosis*

47–67% Cardiac rhabdomyomas

Kidneys
50% Angiomyolipoma*
26% Cystic disease*
2.4% Renal cell carcinoma

Skin
~50% Shagreen patch
~100% Hypopigmented macules*

Nail bed
88% Ungual fibromas

Fig. 12.9: Manifestations of tuberous sclerosis.

OSCE tips 6: Mnemonic for tuberous sclerosis

'ASHLEAF'
Ashleaf spots ('hypopigmented macules'; *Fig. 12.10a*)
Shagreen patches (thick, leathery skin patches in the lumbosacral region; *Fig. 12.10b*)
Heart rhabdomyosarcoma
Lung hamartomas
Epilepsy and cognitive deficits (→ cortical tubers)
Angiomyolipoma of the kidneys
Facial angiofibroma

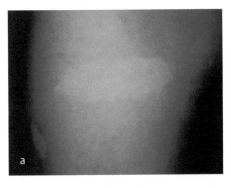 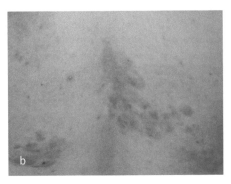

Fig. 12.10: (a) ashleaf spots; (b) shagreen patches indicative of tuberous sclerosis.

Diagnosis and investigation

Ix
- A clinical diagnosis
- Other investigations guided by presentation

DDx
- Infantile spasm (West syndrome)
- Lennox–Gastaut syndrome
- Epilepsy
- Learning disability

Management

- Early involvement of the MDT.
- Family support.
- Identification and management of complications (i.e. AEDs for seizures, surgical excision of intracranial tubers).

Cerebral palsy

Cerebral palsy (CP) is a **non-progressive, permanent** impairment of **motor/postural** development, which arises in the **immature** brain and is often **associated with other abnormalities** (i.e. cognitive, communicative, sensory, behavioural or seizure disorders). It affects 1.2 per 1000 live births.

Pathophysiology

Damage to the immature brain occurring between ~24/40 gestation (prenatal; 75%), birth (perinatal; 10%) and <3 y/o (postnatal; 15%). This results in the following:

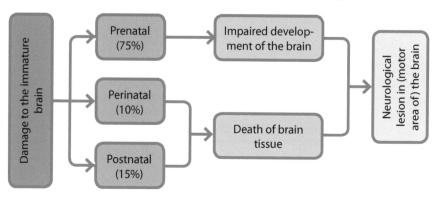

If the lesion affects:

- the motor cortex or pyramidal tracts → upper motor neurone signs (~80%)
- basal ganglia or cerebellum → lower motor neurone signs (~20%).

Clinically, this leads to the following types (*Fig. 12.11*):

1. **Spastic**:
   i. Hemiplegia
   ii. Diplegia
   iii. Quadriplegia

Characterized by upper motor neurone signs:
- Hypertonicity (→ spasticity)
- Hyperreflexia and clonus
- Upgoing plantar reflex ('Babinski')

2. **Dyskinetic** (damage to the basal ganglia):

   i. Athetoid. Characterized by:
      - Abnormal, involuntary, writhing movements (hyperkinesia), mainly affecting the face and extremities
      - Facial grimacing and drooling
      - Feeding and speech impairment
      - Hypotonia
      - Normal reflexes

   ii. Dystonic. Characterized by:
      - Prolonged, slow, repetitive movements, which may affect the whole body region
      - Abnormal posturing
      - Hypotonia
      - Normal reflexes

3. **Ataxic** (damage to the cerebellum). Characterized by:
   - Loss of coordinated muscular contraction → clumsiness, impaired balance and abnormal gait
   - Hypotonia
   - Intention tremor

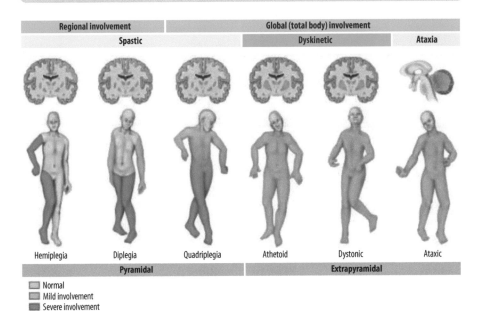

Fig. 12.11: Types of cerebral palsy and areas of brain damage involved.

Epidemiology and risk factors

Prenatal
• Prematurity
• Low birthweight (LBW)
• Twin pregnancy (increases prematurity and LBW)
• Periventricular leukomalacia (see *Section 3.5.4*)
• Intraventricular haemorrhage (see *Section 3.5.4*)
• Chorioamnionitis
• Maternal illness (thyroid disease, seizures, placental disease)

Perinatal
• Asphyxia or other causes of hypoxia (i.e. cardiac arrest)
• LBW
• Neonatal sepsis

Postnatal
• NAI or head trauma
• Infection: meningitis or encephalitis
• Kernicterus
• Seizures

Clinical features

These vary depending on clinical type, with core features described above; however, there are some important generic characteristics that may alert you to the diagnosis of cerebral palsy.

- Delayed developmental milestones (→ head control, crawling, walking)
- Floppiness or stiffness
- Persistence of primitive reflexes
- Feeding or speech abnormalities
- Features of associated disorders (→ seizures, cognitive impairment, learning disability, visual impairment).

Table 12.8: Gait associated with cerebral palsy		
Type	**Gait**	**Description**
Spastic hemiplegia	Circumductive	Unable to flex hip (→ spasticity), so hemipelvis raised and leg swung out to side to allow it to clear the ground. **Walks on tiptoes**.
Spastic diplegia	Scissoring	Spasticity causes adducted, internally rotated hips. **Also walks on tiptoes**.
Ataxic	Ataxic	Broad-based, unsteady and staggering.

Investigation and diagnosis

Hx
- Prenatal, perinatal or postnatal **risk factors**
- Delayed milestones
- Motor abnormalities
- Features of associated conditions
- There is no loss of abilities once achieved – regression is a **Red Flag** for a different diagnosis

Ex
- Motor abnormalities
- Abnormal gait
- Features of associated conditions

Ix
- A clinical diagnosis. Enhanced follow-up for high risk children.
- Functional assessment (GMFCS; see *OSCE tips 7*)

DDx
Broad. It is important to recognize features that indicate a diagnosis **other than CP (NICE 2017, CG62)**:
- **Absence** of risk factors
- Family Hx of progressive neurological disease
- **Loss** of attained abilities
- Development of **focal** neurology
- MRI findings not consistent with diagnosis

Management

Early involvement of the MDT is essential because, as a collective, they can address many of the broad issues that affect children with CP. The main challenges faced by these children and families can be summarized as below:

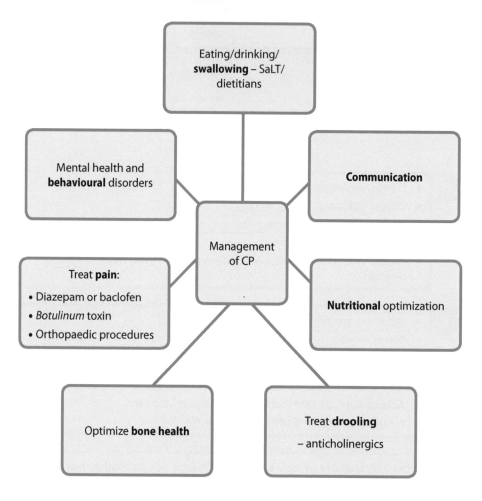

OSCE tips 7: GMFCS

The Gross Motor Function Classification System (GMFCS) is **routinely** used in clinical practice and allows the child's functional abilities to be categorized into 5 levels:

Level I (least affected) → Level V (most affected)

Chapter 13

Musculoskeletal disorders

Leg pain and childhood limp

The limping child is a common case to see in the ED and can present a diagnostic challenge. The DDx is broad and the physician should **bear in mind that sinister pathology and non-accidental injury (NAI)** can present in this way. Here we discuss how to perform a structured assessment of these children and address some common conditions presenting in this way.

Clinical features

Symptoms

HPC

- A thorough pain history is important; however, **referred pain** is common in children, who may describe knee pain despite the pathology coming from the hip.
- **When** is it most severe?
- Any other orthopaedic symptoms (stiffness, clicking, clunking, locking, giving way)?
- Was there trauma? It is possible that the child may not admit to having had an accident.

Systems review

- Any **systemic** features (fevers, rigors, night sweats, ↓weight)?
- Other joints affected?
- Neurological changes?
- GI diseases, such as IBD
- Dermatological diseases, such as psoriasis

Development

- Meeting developmental **milestones? Regression?**

PMH

- Any recent infections?
- Any syndromes?

DH

- Steroids?

Signs

Observations ?febrile ?↑HR

Look

- Watch the child walk ?antalgic ?unable to weight bear
- Leg length discrepancy
- Muscle wasting? Erythema? Swelling? Asymmetry?

Feel

- **Temperature?** Swelling?

Move

- Active and passive range of movement (ROM)

Neurovascular assessment

- Perform a **full neurovascular examination** of the limb

> ### Red Flags
>
> - Worse:
>   - in the morning (→ inflammatory arthropathy)
>   - at night (→ ?malignancy)
> - Systemically **unwell** i.e. night sweats, weight loss (→ malignancy, infection, inflammatory)
> - **Redness** and **swelling** over a joint (→ infection or inflammatory)
> - Unexplained **rashes or bruises** (→ coagulopathy or ?NAI)

Table 13.1: Investigations and examinations for leg pain and childhood limp

Age	Condition	Epidemiology	Pathology	Obs.	Examination	Investigations
>3 years	**Toddler's fracture** (*Fig. 13.1*)	9 months – 3 years of age	Minimally displaced **spiral fractures** of the tibia; **rarely** related to NAI	Normal	Unable to weight bear + tender tibial diaphysis	**Subtle** fracture on radiograph
3–10 years	**Transient synovitis**	Common	Synovial inflammation that **follows an URTI**	Afebrile	Slightly ↓ROM	Mildly raised WCC and ESR; CRP **<20mg/L**
	Perthes' disease (*Fig. 13.2*)	~1 in 1000. 4.5♂:1♀.	Idiopathic avascular necrosis of the femoral head	Afebrile	↓ and internal rotation	Bloods normal; radiograph: sclerosis in femoral head → fragmentation of femoral head → widening and flattening of femoral head; MRI ± bone scan required
10–18 years	**Slipped capital femoral epiphysis (SCFE)** (*Fig. 13.3*)	10 per 100 000. Associated with obesity	Slippage of the proximal femoral growth plate, which may be acute (~20%) or chronic (~80%)	Afebrile	Externally rotated hip ± unable to weight bear (in acute presentation)	Bloods normal; radiographs: **'frog leg'** view required to show subtle slips ± MRI or CT
Any age group	**Fracture**	Common	Usually preceded by history of trauma, although child may not admit it; consider NAI	Normal	Unable to use affected limb + tender fracture site	Fracture on radiograph
	Septic arthritis and osteomyelitis	Incidence in children > adults	Usually due to haematogenous spread of microorganisms or, rarely, penetrating injury; can spread between joint ⇆ bone	Unwell and febrile	↓↓ ROM ± unable to weight bear	↑ **WCC, CRP >20 and ↑ESR** (within 48 hours of onset); effusion on USS; causal organisms described in *Section 13.2.*
	Malignancy	Very rare	Red Flags including night pain and systemic features may be present ± pathological fractures	Afebrile	Reduced ROM ± hepato- or splenomegaly ± regional lymphadenopathy	Radiographs and bone biopsy for diagnosis
	Inflammatory arthropathies	See *Section 13.4*				

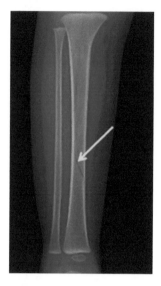

Fig. 13.1: Toddler's fracture.

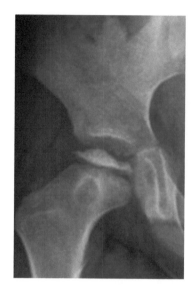

Fig. 13.2: Perthes' disease.

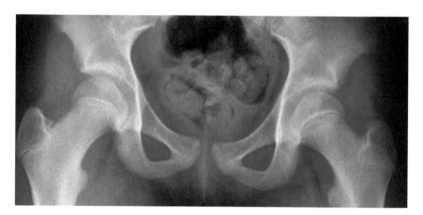

Fig. 13.3: Slipped capital femoral epiphysis.

Investigation and diagnosis

Ix
- Baseline observations
- Bloods inc. CRP (>20mg/L is suggestive of infection) and ESR
- Plain radiographs
- ± disease specific work-up

DDx
- As per *Table 13.1*
- Osgood–Schlatter disease
- Osteochondritis dissecans
- Chondromalacia patellae

Management

Condition	Management
Toddler's fracture	Above-knee cast for 4 weeks
Transient synovitis	NSAIDs and close observation (for septic arthritis)
Perthes' disease	If <6 y/o and <50% of head involved (**'half a dozen, half a head'**) → analgesia, protected weight bearing and physiotherapy, until head re-ossifies If >6 y/o and >50% → operative intervention
SCFE	**Urgent surgical fixation** with cannulated hip screws is indicated in all cases
Fracture	Reduction and immobilization, dependent on the fracture type
Septic arthritis (*Section 13.2.1*)	**Surgical washout** and debridement, with a prolonged course of **antibiotics** Splintage can be used for analgesia for a brief period
Osteomyelitis (*Section 13.2.2*)	Early disease, without septic arthritis, can be trialled with 4–6 weeks of **antibiotics** alone; where this fails, surgical debridement is additionally required

13.2 Bone and joint infections

13.2.1 Septic arthritis

Septic arthritis (SA) is a **surgical emergency**, with prompt diagnosis and management paramount in preventing catastrophic damage to the joint. The hip or knee is affected in 70% of cases and 10% are polyarticular.

Pathophysiology

SA is a bacterial **infection of the synovium**, most commonly due to haematogenous spread ('seeding') from a remote site. Rarely, the cause is direct inoculation (from penetrating injury or surgery) or spread from adjacent osteomyelitis. Joint damage starts to occur after ≥**8 hours**.

Table 13.2: Those affected by SA and the implicated organisms

Patient group	Organism
Neonates	Group B *Strep.*
2–5 year olds	*S. aureus* (most common), HIB, *S. pneumoniae*
Adolescents	*N. gonorrhoeae*
Sickle cell disease	*Salmonella* spp.
Following varicella	Group A (β-haemolytic) *Strep.*

Epidemiology and risk factors

Prematurity (immune function)
Delivered by C-section
Invasive procedures

50% of children affected are <2 years old (*Table 13.2*).

Investigation and diagnosis

Hx
- **Unwell** child with fevers
- Severe joint pain
- In the lower limb → unable to weight bear
- ± Recent infection (→ source of seeding)
- ± Risk factors as above

Ex
- Febrile
- Warm joint ± erythema
- Joint **effusion**
- Joint usually **held in slight flexion**
- Very limited range of motion → **pseudoparalysis**

Ix
- Bloods (↑WCC, CRP >20mg/L, ↑ESR)
- Blood cultures
- Joint **aspiration** – send for MC&S and WCC + RCC
- Radiographs – often **normal** initially
- USS – especially of the hips; show effusion and can guide aspiration
  - N.B. Scan **both** hips in neonates

DDx
- See *Section 13.1*
- Tumours
- Haemarthrosis
- Soft tissue injury

Where practicable, antibiotics should **not be given until after joint aspiration** (i.e. if the child is systemically well with normal observations). This permits MC&S and therefore **targeted antibiotic therapy**.

Management

- Urgent **surgical washout** and debridement + 4–6 weeks of **antibiotics**.

13.2.2 Osteomyelitis

Pathophysiology

An acute **or** chronic bacterial infection of the bone, typically due to haematogenous seeding or, less commonly, penetrating trauma or direct spread from a contiguous joint. Approximately 50% of infections involve the femur or tibia.

The infection tends to affect the **metaphyseal** bone as, at this location, there is sluggish flow of blood through the capillary beds → acute infection. Chronic infection is characterized by the presence of (i) ongoing destruction of bone (a 'sequestrum') and (ii) apposition of newly formed bone (an 'involucrum').

Epidemiology and risk factors

Male preponderance (2.5:1).

Diabetes mellitus
Sickle cell disease
Immunocompromise
Penetrating injury/open fracture

Table 13.3: Those affected by osteomyelitis and the implicated organisms

Patient group	Organism
Neonates	Group B *Strep.*
6 months–3 years	*Kingella kingae*
All ages	*S. aureus* and *S. pneumoniae*
Sickle cell disease	*Salmonella* spp.

Investigation and diagnosis

Hx
- Limb pain
- ± Unable to weight bear
- ± Systemically unwell (often clinically well in chronic osteomyelitis)

Ex
- Overlying erythema and calor
- Tenderness over the affected area
- ± Draining sinus
- Assess ROM of adjacent joint (?contiguous SA)

Ix
- Bloods – ↑WCC, ↑↑↑CRP and ESR
- Blood cultures if unwell
- Radiographs – initially, bone formation; after ~10 days, bone destruction ('osteolysis'), osteopenia and a periosteal reaction (*Fig. 13.4*)
  - in chronic infection → sequestrum and involucrum (*Fig. 13.5*)
- Aspiration ± bone biopsy

DDx
- See *Section 13.1*
- Tumours
- Haemarthrosis
- Soft tissue injury

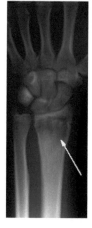

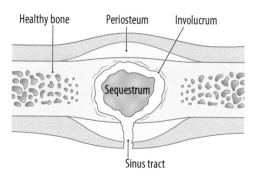

Fig. 13.5: Involucrum in osteomyelitis.

Fig. 13.4: Periosteal reaction in osteomyelitis.

Management

- Initially, **antibiotics** (preferably after aspiration/bone biopsy).
- For chronic or non-responsive infections → surgical debridement.

Paediatric spinal disease is a highly specialist area and a broad understanding is therefore all that is required at an undergraduate level. This chapter concerns adolescent idiopathic scoliosis (AIS) and Scheuermann disease only.

13.3.1 Adolescent idiopathic scoliosis

Anatomy

AIS is an **abnormal lateral curvature** of the spine in the **coronal** plane, with a curve of >10° (→ measured using the Cobb angle (CA); CA = 89° in *Fig. 13.6*).

There is a **major curve** (the largest curve; blue arrow), with a **compensatory curve** (which forms in an attempt to maintain the body's alignment; orange arrow).

Within the major curve, the vertebral bodies also **rotate**, pushing the spinous processes <u>towards</u> the concave side (*Fig. 13.7*).

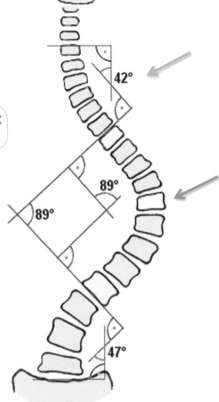

Fig. 13.6: Curvature of spine in scoliosis.

Causes

The aetiologies can be divided into the following:

Structural	Non-structural

• Idiopathic (~70% of all scoliosis cases)
• Congenital
• Neuromuscular
  • neuropathic (e.g. cerebral palsy, spina bifida, tumour)
  • myopathic (e.g. muscular dystrophy)
• Others
  • Marfan disease, Ehlers–Danlos disease and neurofibromatosis
  • traumatic
	• Postural
	  • prolonged poor posture; the scoliosis resolves when the child lies supine
	• Compensatory
	  • the spine is straight, but appears curved due to <u>pelvic</u> obliquity

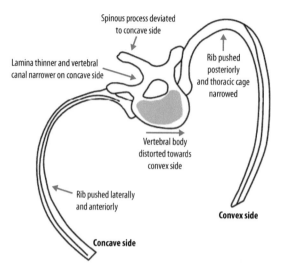

Fig. 13.7: Rotation of vertebral bodies.

Epidemiology and risk factors

Affects children 10–18 years old. Prevalence of ~3%. A **positive family history** is common.

Investigation and diagnosis

Hx
- Classically, AIS is **painless**. A painful scoliosis should prompt work-up for other aetiologies.
- Perceived deformity.

Ex
- Adam's forward bend test → curvature and a **hump on the convex side**.
- A **scoliometer** can be utilized.
- A full neurological exam is required.

Ix
- Radiographs (**note**, these are displayed **as if you are looking at the patient from the back**).
- Measure the Cobb angle (CA).
- ± MRI.

Management

CA <25°	CA 25–45°	CA >45°
Observation and serial radiographs	Bracing until skeletal maturity reached, to reduce further curvature	Spinal fusion

13.3.2 Scheuermann disease

Pathophysiology

Excessive thoracic **kyphosis >45°** due to a defect in secondary ossification within the vertebrae → wedge-shaped vertebral bodies. This leads to **pain** and, over time, an increased likelihood of disc prolapse. Incidence varies; quoted between 0.5 and 8%.

Investigation and diagnosis

Hx
- Back **pain** is common
- Concern about cosmesis

Ex
- Increased kyphosis
- Further increased by bending forwards
- Full neurological assessment required (→ ?prolapsed disc)

Ix
- Radiographs → anterior wedging of vertebrae (*Fig. 13.8*), **Schmorl's nodes** (*Fig. 13.9*), disc narrowing

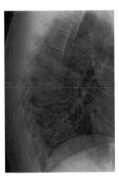

Fig. 13.8: Lateral radiograph of the lumbar spine, demonstrating Scheuermann disease.

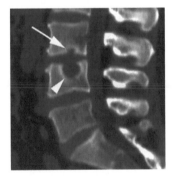

Fig. 13.9: Schmorl's nodes (arrowed): protrusion of the intervertebral disc into the vertebral bodies.

Management

- <60°: observation and physiotherapy
- 60–80°: bracing
- Surgery indicated if: >80°, severe pain or neurological deficit

Rheumatological disorders

Paediatric rheumatology includes a large number of different conditions, all with a broad constellation of symptoms and signs. We provide a broad approach to the work-up of these children and summarize the pertinent findings of the most important conditions.

Investigation and diagnosis

Hx A **comprehensive** history, as detailed in *Chapter 1*, with particular attention paid to:
- The **duration** and **pattern** of joint involvement (?symmetry ?large vs. small joints)
- Morning stiffness and improvement with exercise (→ inflammatory arthropathy)
- A **thorough** review of systems, including eyes, ENT, skin and general features
- Family history (especially JIA, RA, ankylosing spondylitis, IBD and SLE)
- **Impact on function** and schooling

Ex A **comprehensive** examination, as detailed in *Chapter 1*, with particular attention paid to:
- Eyes – conjunctiva and the eyelids
- Nose – nasal mucosa and discharge
- Skin – rashes, nodules, ulcers, hair loss/changes
- Nails – clubbing, ulceration, pitting, onycholysis (*Fig. 13.10*)
- Abdo – hepato- or splenomegaly
- Lymphadenopathy

Ix
- Bloods inc. WCC, ESR, CRP
- Immunological blood tests – ANA, RhF, c-ANCA, p-ANCA, HLA-B27, anticardiolipin Ab
- Joint aspiration
- Radiographs
- ± CT or MRI

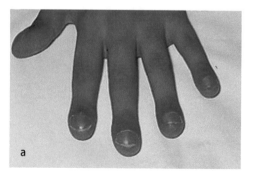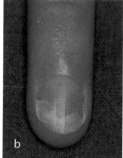

Fig. 13.10: (a) Clubbing; (b) onycholysis.

13.4.1 Juvenile idiopathic arthritis (JIA)

Epidemiology: 1 per 10 000

Pathophysiology: arthritis lasting >**6 weeks and present <16 y/o**. Seven types – 'oligoarthritis' is most common.

Hx: swollen, tender joints (→?limping) with morning stiffness which improves with the day; ± systemic upset (fevers); ± rash (occasionally itchy); ± enthesitis; ± psoriasis (in psoriatic type)

Ex: swollen joint with ↓ ROM; if painful → typically held in mild flexion; ± rash (occasionally itchy); ± enthesitis; ± psoriasis (in psoriatic type)

Ix: ↔/↑ WCC, ↔ /↑ CRP/ESR; ANA+ (70%); RhF+ (polyarthritis type); HLA-B27+ (enthesitis type)

Management: initially, NSAIDs and intra-articular steroid injections for symptom control. Consider PO corticosteroids and/or disease-modifying antirheumatic drugs (DMARDs). Immunomodulators (anti-TNF) used when DMARDs are ineffective.

13.4.2 Systemic lupus erythematosus

Epidemiology: ~1 in 200 000. Female preponderance (4:1). ↑ in Hispanics and African Americans.

Pathophysiology: production of **autoantibodies** against **nuclear antigens** and the formation of **immune complexes**, which lead to tissue injury/organ damage.

Hx: non-specifically unwell (fatigue, fevers, ↓ weight) with pain in multiple joints. Require ≥**4 of the following for diagnosis**:

Ex:

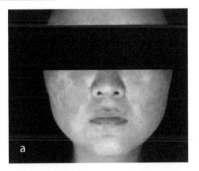
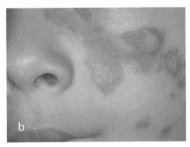

Fig. 13.11: Rash in SLE: (a) malar; (b) discoid.

- Malar rash (*Fig. 13.11a*)
- Discoid rash (*Fig. 13.11b*)
- Photosensitivity
- Oral/nasal ulceration
- Arthritis
- Proteinuria (nephritis)
- Encephalopathy
- Pleuritis or pericarditis
- ↓ RBC/WCC/Plt
- ANA+
- Positive anti-dsDNA/anti-Sm/antiphospholipid Ab

Ix: ↓ WCC and ↓ Plt; ↔ **CRP with ↑ ESR (characteristic)**; low complement (C3/C4); ANA+ (95%); Anti-dsDNA+ (70%); Anti-Sm (35%)

Management: initially, analgesia and NSAIDs; steroids, DMARDs and immunosuppressants are often required.

13.4.3 Juvenile dermatomyositis

Epidemiology: ~2 per 1 million. Female preponderance (5:1).

Pathophysiology: an autoimmune condition causes vasculopathy with subsequent **muscle** and **skin** ischaemia.

Hx: proximal myopathy (∴ difficulty standing/falls) and skin changes (purple discoloration of eyelids – **'heliotrope'** (*Fig. 13.12a*) – and **Gottron papules** – purple papules over extensors, esp. the knuckles (*Fig. 13.12b*). 50% have arthritis. Difficulty swallowing if palatal/pharyngeal muscles affected.

Ix: ↑ CK and LDH (from muscle); ↑ ESR; ANA+ (50%); muscle biopsy; EMG.

Management: steroids started immediately (~6 weeks) + methotrexate. IV immunoglobulin in non-responsive disease.

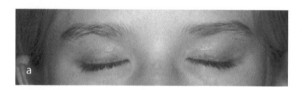 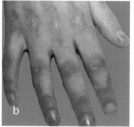

Fig. 13.12: (a) Heliotrope rash; (b) Gottron papules.

13.5 Vitamin D deficiency

A common nutritional deficiency affecting **~10% of young children**, with a slight peak in incidence in teenage years.

Pathophysiology

Synthesized in the skin and activated in the liver and kidney (*Fig. 13.13*), Vitamin D is essential to **calcium and phosphate homeostasis**. Reduced levels lead to ↓ bone **mineralization** ∴ ↓ bone strength. When the growth plates have not fused, this causes **rickets**; thereafter, it causes **osteomalacia**.

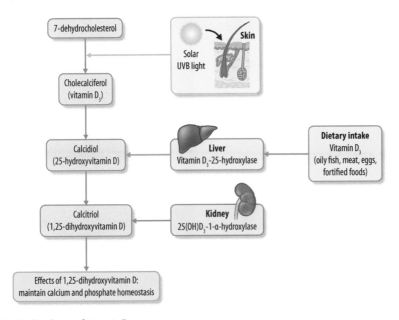

Fig. 13.13: Synthesis of vitamin D.

Risk factors

Inadequate sun exposure
Inadequate dietary intake + veganism
Liver and renal disease (as unable to activate vit D)

Diagnosis and investigation

Hx

Children	Adolescents
• General muscular **aches** • **Weakness** → ± delayed motor milestones • Bowed legs • Short stature	• General muscular **aches** • **Weakness** • **Long bone pain**

 If profoundly hypocalcaemic → tetany and seizures

Ix
- Vitamin D **<25nmol/L**
- ↔ / ↓ Calcium (often normal)
- ↔ / ↓ Phosphate (often normal)
- ↔ / ↑ ALP (high in rickets)
- ↑ PTH
- Radiograph (in rickets) – **splaying** and **fraying of the metaphysis** (*Fig. 13.14*) ± bowing of the legs.

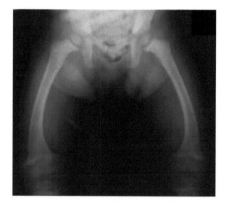

Fig. 13.14: Rickets in a 2-year-old child.

Management

Prevention	↑ safe sun exposure; ↑ vit D in diet (oily fish); ↑ Ca²⁺ intake (milk)
Treatment	Treat the underlying cause; PO vitamin D supplementation
Case finding	Screen the siblings of affected children + offer prevention advice

Genetic disorders

Achondroplasia

Pathophysiology

Affecting ~1:30 000 children, achondroplasia is the most common form of short-limb dwarfism, caused by a mutation in the **fibroblast growth factor receptor-3 (*FGFR3*) gene**. Interestingly, although **autosomal dominant**, ≥80% of cases are due to a *de novo* mutation *in utero*.

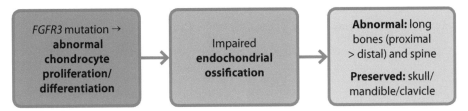

FGFR3 mutation → **abnormal chondrocyte proliferation/ differentiation** → Impaired **endochondrial ossification** → **Abnormal:** long bones (proximal > distal) and spine / **Preserved:** skull/mandible/clavicle

Diagnosis and investigation

Hx
- Normal-sized baby → growth rapidly slows over months
- Delayed motor **milestones**

Ex

Head
- Large relative to body
- Frontal bossing
- Flattened nasal bridge
- Narrowed foramen magnum
- Underdeveloped midface → ear infections ++

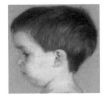

Spine
- Normal trunk
- Thoracic kyphosis
- Lumbar lordosis
- ↑↑ Risk of **spinal stenosis**

Upper limb
- Humerus affected > forearm
- Shortened and broad
- Deep skin creases

Hands
- 'Trident-like' – fingers of equal length and splayed

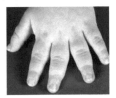

Lower limb
- Thigh affected > leg
- Genu varum
- Broad feet

> **Ix**
> - X-rays: long bones – **flaring**; spine – decreasing interpedicular distance
> - ± MRI (if spinal stenosis)
> - Genetic testing

Management

	Treatment
Teeth	Overcrowding → dentistry
Ears	Prompt treatment of middle ear infections
Spine	Kyphosis: observation; lordosis: observation; lumbar stenosis – ↓ weight, physio ± surgical
Limbs	Genu varum: if progressive → osteotomy; **limb lengthening** may be required if unable to perform ADLs

13.6.2 Osteogenesis imperfecta (OI)

Pathophysiology

An **autosomal dominant** condition with an incidence of 1:20 000. It affects the *COL1A1* and *COL1A2* genes which synthesize **type-1 collagen**: mutations therefore lead to either ↓ **quantity** and/or ↓ **quality**. By considering the roles of type 1 collagen, the features of OI can be deduced:

Bone	Fragility → fractures and progressive deformity (long bones and spinal column)
Teeth	Enamel loss → poor dentition
Ligaments	Hypermobility and joint dislocations
Sclera	Thinning → blue discoloration (secondary to exposure of the choroid)
Cardiac	Aortic incompetence and mitral valve prolapse (both rare)
Ears	Otosclerosis → reduced hearing (common: ~50%)
Skin	Reduced elasticity

There are seven types, of which type I (↓ quantity) and type III (↓ quality) are the most clinically relevant. Type II is rapidly fatal.

Diagnosis and investigation

	Type I	Type III
Bone	• ↑ fractures (possible at birth, but typically occurring thereafter) • Scoliosis (~20%)	• ↑↑↑ fractures (common and multiple at birth) • ↑ deformity leading to **bowing of legs and kyphoscoliosis**
Height	Normal	Reduced due to shortened limbs and curved spine
Teeth	Normal	Translucent; blue or yellow
Ligaments	Hypermobile	Hypermobile
Sclera	Blue	Blue initially; white in childhood
Hearing loss	Common	Common

Ix
- Prenatal USS – for types II and III
- Bloods – usually **normal**
- Radiographs – fractures with excessive callus
- DEXA – to predict risk of fracture in those with less severe disease
- Genetic testing – for formal diagnosis.

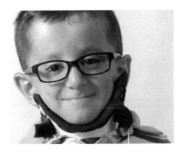

Fig. 13.15: Typical facies seen in OI with a **triangular shape, prominent forehead and small jaw.**

Management

- **Conservative** – physiotherapy to treat weakness and laxity; orthotics for laxity; careful handling
- **Medical** – IV bisphosphonates reduce fracture frequency and improve pain
- **Surgical** – intramedullary nailing is common; correction of kyphoscoliosis.

Chapter 14

Haematological disorders

Iron-deficiency anaemia

Iron deficiency is **the most common cause of anaemia worldwide**. Blood film will show **a microcytic** (small), **hypochromic** (pale) picture of the red blood cells (RBCs).

Pathophysiology

Iron is needed for **haemoglobin production**. Anaemia develops as a result of **insufficient intake** (diet), **insufficient absorption** (chronic inflammation, e.g. Crohn's), or **blood loss** (e.g. menorrhagia).

Epidemiology and risk factors

- Seen in 10% of toddlers and 10% of teenage girls.
- Poor dietary intake (fussy eaters, disadvantaged socio-economic background) at higher risk.

Table 14.1: Risk factors for iron-deficiency anaemia

| Poor dietary intake |
| Chronic inflammatory condition |
| Menorrhagia |
| Lower socio-economic background |

Diagnosis and investigation

Hx
- Often **incidental finding** on blood test and **asymptomatic**.
- If symptomatic – **fatigue**, malaise, poor exercise tolerance, irritability, headache, pre-syncope, **syncope**.
- Comprehensive **dietary** history.
- Pubertal girls – ask about **menstruation**.
- **Systems enquiry** – establish symptoms of possible inflammatory disease or blood loss.

Ex
- **General examination** – pallor, angular stomatitis, glossitis, nail changes, poor weight gain (plot on growth chart).
- **Cardiovascular** – tachycardia, flow murmur.
- **Abdominal** – hepatomegaly/splenomegaly. Indicates haemolysis or infiltration (such as leukaemia) and **should not be seen in iron deficiency**.

Ix
- **Iron studies:** ↓Hb, ↓MCV, ↓ferritin, ↑total iron-binding capacity, ↓transferrin saturation
- **Blood film:** hypochromic, microcytic anaemia (*Fig. 14.1*)

DDx
- Leukaemia
- Other causes of anaemia

Management

- Chronic deficiency is managed with **oral iron replacement** until the haemoglobin is normal and then for another 3 months to ensure stores are replenished.

- **Dietary advice** imperative – green vegetables and red meat contain a lot of iron and it is better absorbed when eaten with vitamin C.

- Blood transfusion is **very rarely** indicated.

- **Failure to respond** to oral iron should trigger **further investigation** into non-dietary causes (malabsorption/blood loss).

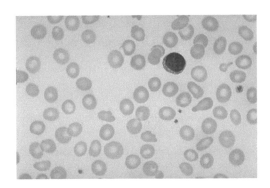

Fig. 14.1: A blood film showing hypochromic, microcytic RBCs in iron deficiency.

Haemolytic anaemia

Anaemia secondary to increased destruction of the erythrocytes. This section covers the common haemolytic anaemias not caused by haemoglobinopathies.

Pathophysiology

- Erythrocyte breakdown happens **intravascularly** (G6PD, autoimmune haemolysis) or **extravascularly** – in the liver and spleen (haemoglobinopathies, membrane defects).
- The result of breakdown is **anaemia**, **splenomegaly**, **hepatomegaly** and unconjugated **hyperbilirubinaemia** (haemoglobin degradation product).
- Haemolysis triggers **reticulocytosis** in the bone marrow. If the marrow cannot compensate for the rate of increased RBC destruction → anaemia.

Epidemiology and risk factors

Condition	Epidemiology	Pathophysiology	Blood film
G6PD deficiency	10–20% Afro-Caribbean, Mediterranean and Middle Eastern males; 1% of females. X-linked.	G6PD prevents damage to RBCs during oxidative stress. Deficiency therefore makes the cells susceptible to damage from oxidation – i.e. if exposed to oxidative drugs or infection.	Fig. 14.2: Heinz bodies (from haem oxidation).
Hereditary spherocytosis	1:5000, autosomal dominant.	Membrane defect that makes RBCs spherical, resulting in destruction by the spleen as they cannot fit through the microvasculature.	Fig. 14.3: Spherocytes (arrows).
Autoimmune haemolytic anaemia	1 in 100 000	Antibodies to red cell membrane lead to their destruction. Often as part of a wider autoimmune process such as SLE or following a viral or *Mycoplasma* infection.	Fig. 14.4: Spherocytes (A) and reticulocytes (B).

Clinical features

Symptoms

- Fatigue, malaise
- Dark urine
- Acute haemolytic crisis – tachycardia, pallor, jaundice, fever

Signs

- Jaundiced sclera
- Splenomegaly ± hepatomegaly
- Gallstones (from bilirubin load)

Table 14.2: Risk factors for haemolytic anaemia

Family history
Afro-Caribbean, Mediterranean or Asian descent.

Investigation and diagnosis

Hx
- **Often asymptomatic**
- During acute haemolytic episode → sudden onset of pallor, jaundice and fever
- **Family history** common
- Ask about **neonatal jaundice** and whether it required treatment
- Ask about recent **infections**, which may trigger haemolysis

Ex
- **Jaundice**, dark urine (but not pale stools), pallor.
- **Splenomegaly**, hepatomegaly.
- Tachycardia and haemodynamic instability (aplastic crisis).

Ix
- FBC, **blood film**, LFTs, coagulation, unconjugated bilirubin, G6PD activity.
- **Coombs test** (positive in autoimmune haemolysis).

DDx
- Aplastic anaemia
- Bone marrow infiltration (leukaemia)

Management

- **Education** – on triggers and signs of acute haemolysis/aplastic crisis.
- **Folic acid supplementation**.
- **Splenectomy** – in severely symptomatic spherocytosis causing growth failure.
- Most post-infectious **autoimmune haemolytic anaemia is self-limiting** and does not require treatment.
- **Parvovirus B19**-induced aplastic crisis usually requires blood transfusion.

OSCE tips 1: Haemolysis triggers

- **Drugs** – nitrofurantoin, quinolones, sulphonamides, antimalarials (G6PD)
- **Infection** – EBV and *Mycoplasma* (autoimmune haemolysis), any serious infection (G6PD)
- **Parvovirus B19** – causes aplastic crisis in spherocytosis
- **Food** – fava (broad) beans (G6PD)

Sickle cell disease

Sickle cell disease (SCD) is an autosomal recessive haemoglobinopathy, often termed HbSS.

Pathophysiology

Amino acid substitution (glutamine → valine) on the beta-globin chain. In low oxygen tension these are prone to **polymerization**, resulting in abnormally shaped ('sickled') red blood cells that (i) obstruct the microcirculation and (ii) are mechanically weak (→ haemolysis). This results in the following:

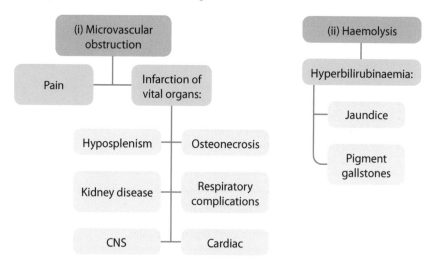

There is a variant termed HbSC, where patients have a less severe form of the disease. Pathologically, the child has one HbS gene and one HbC gene (glutamine → lysine substitution).

Epidemiology and risk factors

1:2000 children in the UK. The main risk factors are **family history, Afro-Caribbean heritage** and living in a **malaria-endemic** country.

Investigation and diagnosis

> **Hx**
> - Fever, pain, lethargy.
> - Recurrent infection.
> - **Symptoms usually do not occur before 6 months of age** as there is sufficient foetal Hb to protect the infant.

Ex
- Pallor/jaundice. Splenomegaly.

Ix
- Bloods (FBC – ↓Hb, ↑reticulocytes, ↓Plt; renal and liver profile annually).
- Blood film – sickle cells and target cells. If asplenic – Howell–Jolly bodies.
- Genetic testing to identify carriers.

DDx
- Thalassaemia
- Pancytopenia
- Sickle cell trait

Sickle cell crisis

There are many different types of sickle cell 'crisis' – a broad term for acute complications of SCD, which are typically **precipitated by infection, cold, hypoxia, dehydration, stress** or **medications**. They are the **most common reason for admission**.

Vaso-occlusive crisis			
Pathophysiology	**Features**	**Investigation**	**Management**
Acute vaso-occlusion of the microvasculature	• Severe pain, which can affect anywhere • ± dactylitis	• Bloods as above • Cross-match • Blood film (sickle and target) Fig. 14.5: Blood film showing sickle (blue arrow) and target (black arrow) cells.	• Identify trigger and treat accordingly (i.e. Abx if infective) • Strong analgesia (often parenteral opioid) • Oxygenation • Keep warm

Acute chest syndrome

Pathophysiology	Features	Investigation	Management
• Acute pulmonary infarct Life-threatening	• Hypoxia • Chest pain • Fever • ± cough	• ABG • Bloods inc. CRP and cultures • CXR – new **pulmonary infiltrates** **Fig. 14.6:** CXR showing new pulmonary infiltrates.	• Empirical antibiotics • Oxygenation • Analgesia • Keep warm • Urgent haematology review ?transfusion • Low threshold for ITU involvement

Management

- These children should be **managed by a haematologist** as they will have ongoing physical and often psychological health needs.
- Due to hyposplenism, **antibiotic prophylaxis** (phenoxymethylpenicillin) is required lifelong.
- **Folic acid** replacement.
- Hydroxyurea (to increase HbF production).
- Some children require regular blood transfusions.
- Bone marrow transplant is curative in 90% but rarely performed.

OSCE tips 2: Complications of sickle cell disease

There are many complications, all of which require very specialist intervention. An appreciation of the following is important, although junior doctors are unlikely to be involved in the management.

In the OSCE, it is useful to ascertain the following:
- **Number of admissions and impact on schooling.**
- **Was diagnosis made prenatally? If not, how did child first present?**
- **Is the child under a regular transfusion programme?**
- **Look for scars – splenectomy or cholecystectomy?**
- **If spleen is palpable, by how many centimetres?**

OSCE tips 2: *(continued)*

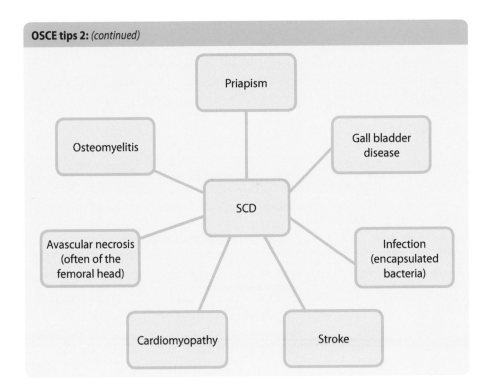

14.4 Thalassaemia

Inherited **defects in haemoglobin synthesis**, affecting either the alpha or beta globin chains. Produces a microcytic, hypochromic anaemia with ineffective erythropoiesis (resulting in a low reticulocyte count) and intravascular haemolysis of abnormal RBCs (resulting in splenomegaly).

Pathophysiology

Normal haemoglobin

- **Foetal Hb (HbF,** $\alpha2\gamma2$). 2 alpha, 2 gamma chains, 75% of Hb at term is HbF and drops to 0% over first 6 months of life.
- **Adult Hb (HbA,** $\alpha2\beta2$). 2 alpha, 2 beta chains, 98% of Hb by 6 months of age.

β-thalassaemia

- Mutations in the **beta globin chains** result in a total absence of normal HbA production (major).
- OR severe reduction in HbA with compensatory higher level of HbF (intermedia).

α-thalassaemia

- Deletion of any of the **4 alpha globin chains**. Deletion of all four means no HbF or HbA can be produced → fatal *in utero* (hydrops fetalis).
- Three chain deletions results in severe anaemia and haemolysis; some HbA can be produced. One or two chain deletions tolerated very well.

Epidemiology and risk factors

- **Alpha thalassaemia** is common in SE Asia, Middle East, India and Africa.
- **Beta thalassaemia** is very common in the Mediterranean with a 1:7 carrier rate in Cyprus.
  - also common in N. Africa, eastern Europe and the Middle East.
- **15 million** people worldwide have **clinically significant thalassaemia**, with many millions more as carriers.

Table 14.3: Risk factors for thalassaemia

Family history
Mediterranean, Middle Eastern, Indian descent
Cypriot (β-thalassaemia major)

Clinical features – variable (see *Table 14.4*)

Table 14.4: Clinical features of thalassaemia

Disease	Genotype	Clinical picture	Findings on blood film
β-thalassaemia major (Cooley's anaemia)	Homozygous β⁰-thalassaemia (no normal beta chains)	• Severe haemolysis and ineffective erythropoiesis make child transfusion-dependent • Hepatosplenomegaly • Iron overload (from transfusions and consequence of thalassaemia)	• Severe anaemia • Severe microcytosis and hypochromasia • Show anisocytosis (unequal cell size) and fragmented RBCs
β-thalassaemia intermedia	Compound heterozygous β⁰- and β⁺-thalassaemia	• Less severe haemolysis so not transfusion-dependent • Will have large splenomegaly • Iron overload	• Moderate anaemia • Moderate microcytosis
β-thalassaemia minor	Heterozygous β⁰- and β⁺-thalassaemia	• Asymptomatic	• Mild anaemia • ± Mild microcytosis • Low reticulocyte count
Silent carrier	α-/αα	• Asymptomatic	• Normal full blood count and film
α-thalassaemia trait (minor)	αα/-- (type 1) α-/α- (type 2)	• Usually asymptomatic	• Mild anaemia • ± Mild microcytosis • Low reticulocyte count
Haemoglobin H (α-thalassaemia intermedia)	α-/--	• Mild jaundice and splenomegaly from haemolysis of abnormal RBCs	• Mild–moderate microcytic anaemia • Heinz bodies
Hydrops fetalis (α-thalassaemia major)	--/--	• Congestive cardiac failure *in utero* → fatal *in utero* or soon after birth • Cannot make any normal haemoglobin (HbF or HbA)	• Severe anaemia

Hx
- Symptoms manifest at age **6–12 months** as the foetal haemoglobin level drops.
- **Microcytic, hypochromic anaemia that does not respond to iron supplements**, especially in a child from a high prevalence ethnic background.
- **Failure to thrive** and growth failure.

Ex
- **Splenomegaly, hepatomegaly** (in major disease), variable **jaundice, pallor**.
- **Growth failure** and heart failure (beta thalassaemia major).
- **Ineffective erythropoiesis** – osteopenia, bone deformity (frontal bossing and dental malocclusion), pathological fractures from excessive metabolic energy expenditure.
- **Iron overload** – iron deposits cause hepatic cirrhosis, cardiomyopathy and diabetes (pancreatic deposits).
- Long-term IV access for transfusion-dependent children (Port-A-Cath).

Investigation and diagnosis

Ix
- FBC ($\downarrow$ Hb, $\downarrow$ reticulocytes), LFTs ($\uparrow$ bilirubin), iron studies ($\uparrow$ iron level).
- Blood film (microcytic, hypochromic anaemia).
- **Hb electrophoresis** is diagnostic and quantifies amount of HbF, HbA and HbA2.

DDx
- Anaemia of chronic disease
- Anaemia of renal failure
- Iron-deficiency anaemia

Management

Disease	Management
β-thalassaemia major	• Regular (monthly) **transfusions** • **N.B. High risk of antibody development; this makes finding compatible blood challenging** • May need long-term access for transfusions, which is an infection risk • Iron **chelation** (see below) • Bone marrow transplant is curative
β-thalassaemia/α-thalassaemia minor (carriers)	• **No treatment** required • Advice should be given on risk to future children if partner also from high risk background
α-thalassaemia major (hydrops fetalis)	• **Fatal** *in utero*/soon after birth unless receive *in utero* transfusions, then will need them for life
α-thalassaemia intermedia (HbH disease)	• Anaemia is significant and **may need transfusions** but less frequently • Iron overload is still a significant risk and children need close monitoring
Iron overload	• **Oral chelation** therapy should be started before organ damage of iron deposits starts (age 2–3) • Regular monitoring of potential end organ damage (growth, cardiomyopathy, hepatic and pancreatic function)

X-linked recessive clotting factor deficiency resulting in increased bleeding risk. May be classed as mild (5–25% of normal factor levels), moderate (1–4% of normal) or severe (<1%).

Pathophysiology

- **Reduction or absence of factor VIII** (haemophilia A) **or IX** (haemophilia B)
- FVIII and FIX are part of the intrinsic **coagulation pathway** (*Fig. 14.7*)
- Clots are unable to form:
  - → **Spontaneous bleeding** (severe disease)
  - → **Poor haemostasis** after minimal trauma (presentation of mild–moderate disease).

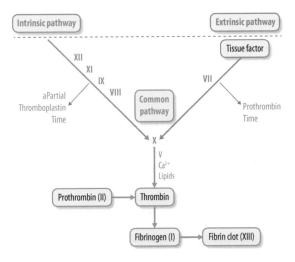

Fig. 14.7: Coagulation cascade.

Epidemiology and risk factors

- Haemophilia A (FVIII deficiency) 1:5000.
- Haemophilia B (Factor IX deficiency, aka Christmas disease) 1:30 000.
- Both X-linked but females can occasionally be mildly affected.

Table 14.5: Risk factors for haemophilia
Male sex
Family history

Clinical features

Symptoms
- Excessive bleeding from minor trauma
- Spontaneous bleeding:
  - Haemarthroses pathognomonic

- Muscular haematomas
- Epistaxis
- Intracerebral bleeds (in severe disease).
- Impaired/limited mobility due to joint involvement.

Signs
- Chronic joint damage
- Difficult vascular access → may need long-term vascular access

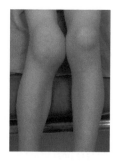

Fig. 14.8: Acute haemarthrosis of the right knee in a boy with haemophilia A.

Investigation and diagnosis

Hx	• Spontaneous bleeding or excessive bleeding after minimal trauma; **moderate disease often presents in toddlers as they learn to walk.**
	• Severe disease may present in the **newborn period** as an **intracerebral bleed**, or bleeding post-circumcision in some ethnic groups.
	• There will be **family history in 2/3** cases.

Ex	• **Spontaneous haemarthroses are pathognomonic of haemophilia.**
	• Examine for joint and muscle swellings and bruises.
	• Look for long-term access and scars of previous access/surgeries. Make sure you **examine the head for neurosurgical scars.**

Ix	• **Bloods** (FBC, coagulation, factor levels, fibrinogen, LFTs). **APTT will be prolonged.**
	• Prenatal diagnosis can be offered in those with a family history.

DDx	• von Willebrand disease
	• Vitamin K deficiency
	• DIC or liver failure

Management

- Haemophilia A → recombinant factor VIII.
- Haemophilia B → recombinant factor IX.
- Keeping levels at 2% of normal should prevent most bleeds and significantly reduces the rate of haemophilia-related arthropathy.
- Prophylaxis typically begins at 2–3 years of age but may be needed earlier in severe disease.

- If the child bleeds acutely the level should be increased; in life-threatening bleeds (such as intracerebral bleeds) or if they need surgery levels need to be 100% and kept >30% to minimize the risk of further bleeding.
- NSAIDs, aspirin and IM injections are contraindicated.

OSCE tips 3: Long-term IV access

Children with severe haemophilia often need **daily/weekly injections** of the factor they are deficient in → long-term access is required, usually with a **tunnelled central venous catheter** (such as a **Hickman line** or **Port-A-Cath** (*Fig. 14.9*)).

This can be **antiseptically accessed at home** to allow the family independence.

Complications:

- infection
- can stop working or become blocked
- needs replacing as child grows
- requires general anaesthetic for insertion

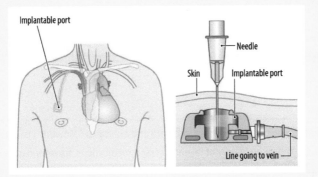

Fig. 14.9: Port-A-Cath.

14.6 Thrombocytopenia

Reduced platelet number (**<150** × **10⁹**): in children, this is most commonly due to idiopathic thrombocytopenic purpura (**ITP**), which this section discusses.

Pathophysiology

- Broadly, may be due to ↓ **production** (i.e. bone marrow failure, hereditary syndromes and medication) or ↑ **destruction** (i.e. ITP, TTP, HUS, DIC) – the aetiologies are very broad, however.
- ITP pathophysiology can be summarized as:

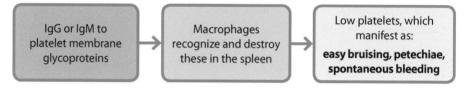

| IgG or IgM to platelet membrane glycoproteins | → | Macrophages recognize and destroy these in the spleen | → | Low platelets, which manifest as: **easy bruising, petechiae, spontaneous bleeding** |

Epidemiology and risk factors

~4:100 000 children. Onset approximately 2–10 years of age and usually **1–4 weeks after a viral illness**.

Diagnosis and investigation

Hx
- **Sudden onset** of **petechiae**, **purpura** and **epistaxis** following a viral infection.
- Take a thorough history of recent illnesses, medications, travel and general symptoms.
- **ITP is a diagnosis of exclusion**.

Ex
- **Bloods – FBC**, coagulation, blood film. In ITP the **white cell** and **red cell count** will be **normal** (unlike in bone marrow disease).
- **Bone marrow aspirate** if unsure of diagnosis/atypical features, to rule out leukaemia or aplastic anaemia.

Ix
- **Purpura** (*Fig. 14.10*) and **petechiae** (rarely present if platelets >20×10⁹).
- **Hepatosplenomegaly** may be present (but should make you suspicious of non-ITP-mediated cause)
- Be confident you have ruled out other causes before diagnosing ITP – is there any **evidence of sepsis** or **non-accidental injury (NAI)**?

DDx
- NAI
- Leukaemia
- Aplastic anaemia
- HSP
- DIC
- Meningococcal sepsis

Management

- ITP is usually **self-limiting** and **no treatment** needed.
- Oral **steroids** or **IV immunoglobulin (IVIG)** may be used in children with significant bleeding, but side-effects are significant.
- Platelet transfusions are only indicated if life-threatening, as antibodies will destroy any transfused platelets.
- **Parents should be given advice** about management of risk.
- **Avoid contact sports**.

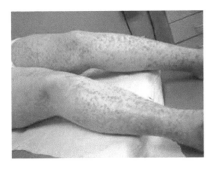

Fig. 14.10: A child with multiple purpura secondary to ITP.

Chapter 15

Dermatological disorders

Congenital and newborn

15.1.1 Infantile haemangioma

Epidemiology: these lesions are present in ~3–5% of infants and typically manifest before 4 weeks of age.

Pathophysiology: they are **benign** vascular tumours and represent 7% of all benign tumours of infancy. They can be broadly grouped into capillary (superficial) and cavernous (deep).

Distribution: usually found in the **head and neck**.

- Capillary: they are red macules or papules, with a **'strawberry'**-like appearance (*Fig. 15.1*).
- Cavernous: appear as **bluish, nodular** swellings (*Fig. 15.2*).

Management: most will spontaneously involute; however, corticosteroids, propranolol and imiquimod may be used to induce this.

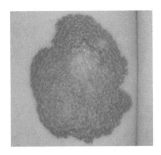

Fig. 15.1: Capillary haemangioma.

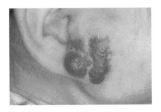

Fig. 15.2: Cavernous haemangioma.

15.1.2 Mongolian blue spot

Epidemiology: these are **congenital** lesions commonly found in *African, Asian and Hispanic* children.

Pathophysiology: they are due to entrapment of melanocytes in the dermis.

Distribution: typically found in the **lumbar and sacral** areas.

Appearance: they are **blue–black macules** (*Fig. 15.3*) which *may be confused with bruising*.

Management: treatment is not required and most will spontaneously regress, fading slowly in the early years.

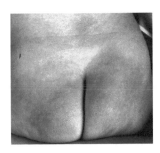

Fig. 15.3: Mongolian blue spot affecting the sacral area.

15.1.3 Café au lait spot

Epidemiology: these macules are present in up to **20% of black children** and, less commonly, in Caucasians. In some instances, *they are associated with neurofibromatosis* (type 1) and McCune–Albright syndrome.

Pathophysiology: they are due to high melanin content in the skin.

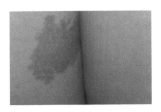

Fig. 15.4: The macular, pale brown appearance of café au lait (coffee with milk) spots.

Distribution: they may be found anywhere on the skin, but often on the buttocks.

Appearance: they are **pale brown macules** (*Fig. 15.4*).

Management: they do not require medical care but, **if the child develops ≥6 by 5 years old, neurofibromatosis type 1 should be considered**.

15.1.4 Erythema toxicum neonatorum (ETN)

Epidemiology: ETN (aka 'neonatal urticaria') occurs in **up to one-third of all neonates**, usually within the first 2 weeks of life.

Pathophysiology: their aetiology is not clear.

Distribution: the rash is primarily found on the trunk and buttocks (*Fig. 15.5*), but may spread elsewhere.

Appearance: the lesions are erythematous, **blanching** macules. Importantly, there is an *absence of any other symptoms*.

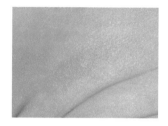

Fig. 15.5: ETN affecting the abdomen of a neonate.

Management: reassurance is all that is required; they usually disappear in weeks/months.

15.1.5 Milia

Epidemiology: these skin lesions are seen in up to 50% of infants, but may affect older children too.

Pathophysiology: they are benign epidermal inclusion cysts.

Distribution: they occur in clusters, often around the eyes, cheeks, lips and chin (*Fig. 15.6*).

Appearance: they are **white–yellow nodules** and measure only a couple of mm in diameter.

Management: no treatment is usually required; they usually disappear in weeks/months.

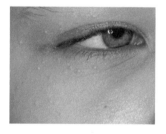

Fig. 15.6: Milia in a child.

15.1.6 Capillary malformation ('port wine stain')

Epidemiology: occurs in <0.5% of newborns; usually **idiopathic**.

Pathophysiology: congenital vascular malformations in the superficial vessels of the dermis, that *enlarge as the child grows* and *do not regress with age*.

Distribution: most capillary malformations involve the face, with around 50% crossing the midline.

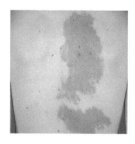

Fig. 15.7: Port wine stain affecting right hand side of back, which does not cross midline.

Appearance: macular, well-defined patches that are red/purple in colour. They are therefore often referred to as **'port wine stains'**.

Management: laser treatment can help to improve the cosmetic appearance.

Sturge–Weber syndrome

This is a rare disorder that is found in about 10% of children that have a port wine stain affecting the distribution of the ophthalmic branch of the trigeminal nerve. However, in addition to affecting the dermis, the vascular malformations affect the ipsilateral meninges (arachnoid and pia) and cerebral cortex. The effect of this varies in affected children but may include: learning difficulties and developmental delay, seizures (which progress from focal to generalized and get worse despite treatment), hemiparesis, macrocephaly and glaucoma/visual loss.

15.2 Bacterial infections

15.2.1 Scarlet fever

Epidemiology: scarlet fever is a **notifiable** disease that usually affects children between 5 and 10 years of age.

Pathophysiology: it is due to infection with group A β-haemolytic streptococci (**S. pyogenes**). This is typically of the throat, but may also be of surgical sites, the uterus or the skin (cellulitis).

History: prodrome: pharyngitis, fever and myalgia.

Within 1 week, the characteristic features appear and include:

- 'Scarlatiniform rash' (*Fig. 15.8a*) – appears on the neck, chest and axillae. The rash is punctate and erythematous, with a **'sandpaper'-like** texture
- Circumoral pallor (*Fig. 15.8b*) – there is notable pallor around the mouth
- White strawberry tongue (*Fig. 15.8c*)
- Pastian's lines – confluent petechiae in the axillae and groin creases.

Appearance: after ~7–10 days, desquamation is commonly seen on the skin of the face, palms and fingers.

Investigation and diagnosis: diagnosis can be definitively made with a **throat swab**.

Management: treatment is with **penicillin** for 10/7.

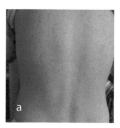 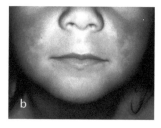 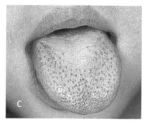

Fig. 15.8: Scarlet fever: (a) scarlatiniform rash on back; (b) circumoral pallor; (c) strawberry tongue.

15.2.2 Impetigo

Epidemiology: impetigo is the most common bacterial infection of the skin that may be seen at any age, but is especially common ≤4 years old.

Pathophysiology: the organisms responsible are primarily **S. aureus or S. pyogenes**. These are inoculated into the skin through a break, with lesions typically occurring 7–14 days later.

History: there are two common forms:

- Non-bullous (*Fig. 15.9a*): multiple vesicles or pustules appear on exposed regions of skin, usually the face or limbs. These **easily rupture and leave a 'honey-coloured' crust,** which may be pruritic and excoriated.
- Bullous (*Fig. 15.9b*): this is most often seen in **neonates**. Thin, **friable** bullae appear and readily rupture, leaving an erythematous base with a scaly collarette.

Investigations: diagnosis is usually clinical.

Management: treatment is with a **topical antibiotic** (such as fusidic acid). Gentle cleaning of the lesions is recommended and, if the rash is pruritic, topical antihistamine is of value.

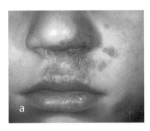 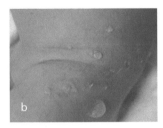

Fig. 15.9: Impetigo: (a) non-bullous; (b) bullous.

Viral infections

Chickenpox (varicella)

Epidemiology: chickenpox is a **highly contagious** infection that affects most children (≥90%) before their teenage years.

Pathophysiology: varicella zoster virus (VZV) is the causal organism. It initially colonizes the respiratory tract, before spreading to the reticuloendothelial system, viscera and skin.

History: there is a preceding viral **prodrome** (mild fever, headache, malaise). After ~10–14 days, the classical rash appears on the **face, neck and trunk** (*Fig. 15.10a*) with *relative sparing* of the limbs.

Appearance: the rash is **pruritic**. It begins as papules, before evolving to vesicles and pustules, which then crust over (*Fig. 15.10b*).

Management: diagnosis is clinical and treatment should be symptomatic, with paracetamol for fever and antihistamines for pruritus. During their contagious period, these children should **stay away from neonates, pregnant women and the immunocompromised**. The child is infective from a few days before the rash appears, and may return to school 5 days after the lesions **appear**.

> **Complications:** CNS – encephalitis, meningitis; bacterial infection – impetigo, pneumonia, myocarditis.

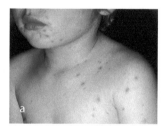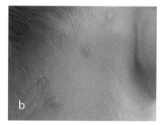

Fig. 15.10: Chickenpox: (a) distribution; (b) appearance.

Measles

Epidemiology: transmitted via airborne respiratory droplets, measles is a **very highly contagious** *notifiable* **disease**. Although vaccinated for routinely in the UK, cases are still seen.

Pathophysiology: *Morbillivirus* replicates in the respiratory tract before disseminating to the lymphatics, viscera and skin.

History: a **prodrome** of high fever (>40°C), rhinorrhoea, cough and diarrhoea is often seen.

Appearance: the **'morbilliform' rash** appears on the head and neck (*Fig. 15.11a*), which spreads to the trunk and then the limbs. The rash begins as erythematous macules and papules, which become confluent over a few days. Classically, the child will have

Koplik spots (*Fig. 15.11b*) that are found opposite the upper 2nd molars and look like a white speck ('grain of rice') on a red base.

Management: a **salivary swab** is required for diagnosis, and management is much the same as for chickenpox, using supportive measures only. Children are contagious for ~4 days before the rash appears and ~4 days after.

 Complications: otitis media, diarrhoea, pneumonia and, rarely, encephalitis.

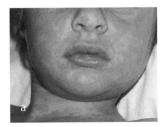 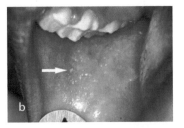

Fig. 15.11: Measles: (a) morbilliform rash; (b) Koplik spots (arrow) on tongue.

15.3.3 Rubella

Epidemiology: rubella is an exceptionally rare infection caused by **Rubivirus** that is transmitted via respiratory droplets.

Pathophysiology: the virus initially invades the respiratory tract before replicating in the reticuloendothelial system. Thereafter, there is widespread dissemination.

History: there may be a viral **prodrome** present, although this is less common in young children.

Appearance: on examination, there is often **lymphadenopathy** present. The rash, which is a

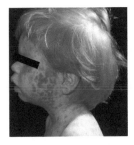

Fig. 15.12: Classical maculopapular rash of rubella, initially affecting child's face.

red-pink maculopapular rash, **begins on the face** (*Fig. 15.12*) before spreading to the trunk and limbs, much like measles. It typically fades after 3 days.

Management: salivary samples are taken for diagnosis and treatment is supportive. Children are infective for up to 4 days after symptoms appear.

OSCE tips 1: Complications of congenital infections

Rubella: deafness, congenital heart disease and cataracts, especially if infected <8 weeks' gestation.
Cytomegalovirus (CMV): cerebral palsy, epilepsy, deafness.
Varicella zoster: if contracted in the first half of pregnancy, infection can cause severe scarring, digital dysplasia and ocular and neurological defects.

15.3.4 Fifth disease ('slapped cheek' or erythema infectiosum)

Epidemiology: spread via respiratory droplets, up to 60% of the population is infected with the causal virus, ***Parvovirus B19***, by adulthood. Unusually for childhood infections, *peak incidence is in the spring and summer months*.

Pathophysiology: the symptoms of fifth disease are thought to be due to deposition of IgM in the skin, formed by a Th1-mediated response to the virus.

History: prodromal symptoms are usually seen and last a few days only. This is characteristically followed by a **period of 7–10 days** in which the child is free of symptoms.

Appearance: the classical erythematous rash then appears on the cheeks, with obvious **sparing of the nose, philtrum, mouth and eyes** (*Fig. 15.13a*). This lasts ~2–4 days and is followed by the development of a **maculopapular ('lacy') rash on the extensor surfaces** (*Fig. 15.13b*).

Management: diagnosis is usually clinical and management is symptomatic; however, note that in children with haemolytic diseases (such as sickle cell), there is **a risk of aplastic anaemia** development.

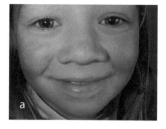 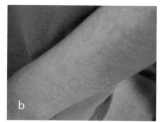

Fig. 15.13: Fifth disease: (a) sparing of nose, philtrum, mouth and eyes; (b) lacy rash on extensor surface of forearm.

15.3.5 Molluscum contagiosum

Epidemiology: this common condition caused by **molluscum contagiosum virus** – a member of the pox family – is spread by direct contact and *often causes outbreaks* in schools.

Pathophysiology: it infects only the epidermis, where it produces lobulated lesions.

Distribution: lesions are on the **trunk and extremities** of children, where they are usually **clustered** together.

Appearance: domed, flesh-coloured papules with a central umbilication, measuring 2–5 mm (*Fig. 15.14*).

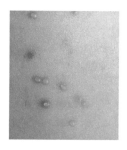

Fig. 15.14: Molluscum contagiosum: fleshy papules with central umbilication.

Management: diagnosis is clinical and lesions will generally resolve spontaneously within 18 months. Children should **avoid scratching** (as auto-inoculation is possible or it may introduce secondary bacterial infection) **and towel sharing**, but are otherwise not restricted.

15.3.6 Hand, foot and mouth disease

Epidemiology: *not to be confused with 'foot and mouth disease'*, this disease is caused by **Coxsackie virus** and spread predominantly by the faeco-oral route. It is seen in infants and those under ~10 years of age.

Distribution: a viral **prodrome** is often seen, causing fever, malaise and a sore mouth. Thereafter, lesions **appear in the mouth, hands** (palms and between the fingers) **and soles**.

Appearance: lesions in the mouth begin as **erythematous macules**, which develop into vesicles before eroding and leaving a **yellow ulcer** (*Fig. 15.15a*). On the palms and soles, lesions follow a similar sequence, but are typically white–grey in colour, with surrounding erythema (*Fig. 15.15b*).

Management: diagnosis is clinical and treatment is supportive. If mouth lesions are causing distress, topical analgesia (such as lidocaine gel) may be applied.

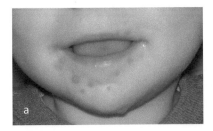 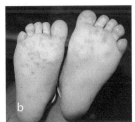

Fig. 15.15: Hand, foot and mouth disease: (a) erythematous macules with yellow ulceration; (b) typical appearance of pedal rash.

15.3.7 Common wart

Epidemiology: common 'viral' warts are caused by **human papillomavirus (HPV)** and are seen in ≤20% of school-age children.

Distribution: although they may affect anywhere, common warts are most common on the hands of children.

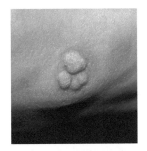

Appearance: discrete flesh-coloured papular lesions with a **rough, hyperkeratotic surface** (*Fig. 15.16*).

Fig. 15.16: A cluster of common warts.

Management: diagnosis is clinical and treatment is dependent on patient preference. Where treatment is requested, **topical salicylic acid** is indicated in the first instance, although cryotherapy is useful for multiple warts.

Pathophysiology: tinea is a **fungal infection** caused by the dermatophytes genera, which induces a delayed (type IV) hypersensitivity reaction.

Distribution: tinea only affects the **keratinized layer** of the skin. It is classified based on the anatomical location that it affects: head (**'capitis'**), trunk ('corporis', aka **'ringworm'**), groin (**'cruris'**) or feet (**'pedis'**). In children, tinea capitis is the most common fungal infection.

Appearance:
- Capitis (*Fig. 15.17a*): the rash causes scaling of the scalp ± localized alopecia
- Corporis (*Fig. 15.17b*): a well-circumscribed, erythematous and scaly lesion, with an area of central clearing
- Cruris: most often seen in males, this is a well-defined, red-brown macular lesion that may contain vesicles or pustules
- Pedis: this is commonly referred to as 'athlete's foot'.

Investigation and diagnosis: diagnosis can be made via microscopic examination of a **skin scraping**.

Management: treatment is usually with **topical antifungal** agents (such as clotrimazole) with the exception of tinea corporis, which is treated with oral agents (terbinafine) for up to 6 weeks.

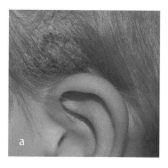 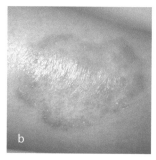

Fig. 15.17: (a) tinea capitis with resultant localized alopecia; (b) tinea corporis showing a well-circumscribed lesion.

Epidemiology: although not especially common in the UK, **outbreaks** do occasionally occur in schools.

Pathophysiology: transferred through prolonged skin-to-skin contact, the *Sarcoptes scabiei hominis* mite is an obligate **human** parasite. Mites live and lay their eggs in the stratum corneum, which mounts a **type IV hypersensitivity** reaction to the mites, eggs and faeces.

Distribution: the major sites for infection are the face, neck, hands (particularly web spaces) and soles of the feet.

Appearance: the lesions cause an **intractable itching**, often worse at night. Lesions are **erythematous papules** (*Fig. 15.18a*), and are associated with **'burrows'** (*Fig. 15.18b*) – thready, grey elevations that represent the movement of the hatching larvae.

Investigation and diagnosis: the diagnosis is usually clinical but, where there is uncertainty, a **scraping** can be viewed under the microscope.

Management: all of the patient's **close contacts** should be treated concurrently and close contact avoided. First-line management is with **permethrin**, which is applied to the whole body. The pruritus is particularly troublesome, but **antihistamine** may help in some cases. All clothes, bedlinen and towels should be **washed on a hot cycle**.

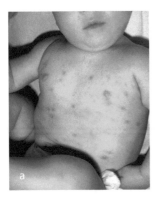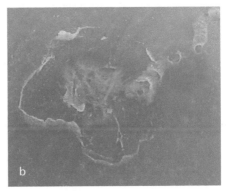

Fig. 15.18: Scabies: (a) papules; (b) burrows. The scabies mite travelled towards the upper right and can be seen at the end of the burrow.

Inflammatory conditions

15.5.1 Atopic eczema

Although a variety of eczematous conditions exist, atopic eczema (synonymous with 'atopic dermatitis') is the most common type in children. Its characteristic appearance and history are easily recognized, although the **location of the rash varies with age**.

Pathophysiology

- Atopic eczema is a **chronic inflammatory condition** of the skin.
- Following a sensitizing event – with current evidence supporting the 'hygiene hypothesis' – the immune system mounts a Th2-mediated response to irritants/allergens, with overexpression of IL-4, IL-5 and IL-13.
- Triggers can be varied but may include:
  - stress or pregnancy
  - environmental irritants such as detergents, fabrics, food, mites, animal dander, and extremes of temperature.
- This causes an acutely pruritic lesion that, over time (and particularly if children scratch), can become chronic and lichenified (thick and leathery).

Epidemiology and risk factors

- Up to **20% of children** have some degree of atopic eczema and most **present before the age of 5 years**.

Table 15.1: Risk factors for atopic eczema
Family history of atopic eczema
Personal history of allergic rhinitis
Personal history of asthma

Clinical features

Distribution

- Varies depending on the child's age:
  - infants: **cheeks** (*Fig. 15.19a*) and scalp
  - mobile infant: as above, plus the extensor surfaces
  - older children: **flexures** (antecubital (*Fig. 15.19b*) and popliteal fossae (*Fig. 15.19c*)), wrists and ankles.

Signs

- Atopic eczema is a pruritic, poorly defined erythematous lesion associated with dry skin.
  - in acute exacerbations, vesicles may appear and the lesions are often excoriated due to pruritus
  - chronically, the lesions may become thickened and leathery (**lichenification**) (*Fig. 15.19d*).
- Particular care should be taken to look for **secondary bacterial infection**, suggested by the presence of pustules or crusting and, in severe cases, systemic symptoms.

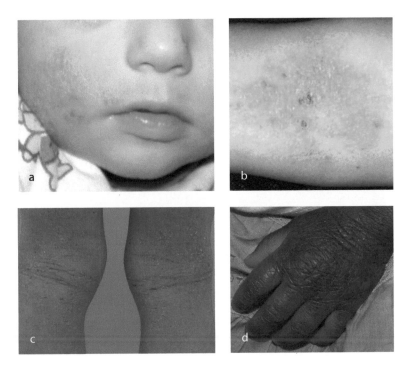

Fig. 15.19: Eczema, affecting: (a) cheeks in infants; (b) antecubital fossae and (c) popliteal fossae in older children; (d) lichenification.

Investigation and diagnosis

> **Ix**
> - Formal diagnostic procedures are not normally required.
> - The severity of eczema may be formally assessed using a validated rating tool, such as the Patient-Oriented Eczema Measure (POEM) or a simple visual analogue scale.

Diagnostic criteria (NICE 2007, CG57)

Itchy skin, plus ≥3 of:
- Flexural involvement
- History of dry skin in last year
- Personal or family history of hay fever or asthma
- If child now older, a previous history of cheek or flexural dermatitis
- If child now >4 y/o, onset of symptoms ≤2 y/o.

Management

- **Identify trigger factors** and manage them appropriately.
- The mainstay of treatment, even when there is no acute lesion present, is **consistent application of emollient to the whole body**. Emollients should also be used to replace the child's usual soap.
- Oral antihistamines are not offered routinely, but can be given where pruritus is significant.
- The remaining treatments **are based on the severity** of the lesion (see *Table 15.2*).

Table 15.2: Stepped approach for managing atopic eczema	
Mild	• Mild potency topical corticosteroids
Moderate	• Moderate potency topical corticosteroids • Topical calcineurin inhibitors (tacrolimus or pimecrolimus)
Severe	• High potency topical corticosteroids • Topical calcineurin inhibitors (tacrolimus or pimecrolimus) • ± Phototherapy (under dermatologist's care only) • ± Systemic therapy (under dermatologist's care only)

15.5.2 Henoch–Schönlein purpura

Henoch–Schönlein purpura (HSP) is a systemic, **small vessel vasculitis** that peaks between the ages of 4 and 6.

Pathophysiology

- HSP is an autoimmune IgA-mediated vasculitis. **IgA is deposited in the target organs** (skin, GI tract, kidneys and joints), causing an inflammatory reaction.
- It is often **triggered** by a preceding streptococcal throat infection (*S. pyogenes*).

Epidemiology and risk factors

- There is an incidence of ≤20 per 100 000 people, mainly affecting those aged 3–15 years.
- Due to its association with streptococcal infection, it is more common in winter.

Table 15.3: Risk factors for HSP
Male sex (2:1)
Preceding streptococcal infection

Clinical features

OSCE tips 2: The tetrad of HSP

1. **Palpable purpuric rash**
   - A rash on the buttocks and/or extensor surface of the legs is nearly always present
2. **Arthralgia**
   - Arthralgia is common and typically affects the lower limb
3. **Abdominal pain**
   - Abdominal pain ± nausea is present in about half of children. 2–3% of children may develop intussusception and there may be (bloody) diarrhoea
4. **Renal involvement**
   - A variety of symptoms due to renal involvement may be present, such as haematuria, nephrotic syndrome (proteinuria, hypoalbuminaemia and generalized oedema) or acute kidney injury

---

Signs

- On inspection, patients appear mildly unwell and may be febrile. They commonly have a **symmetrical macular rash** that, within a day, evolves into **palpable purpuric papules** (*Fig. 15.20*) (which may coalesce, *resemble bruising*) *and do not blanch.*

- Inspect for swollen, tender joints.

- Palpate the abdomen for any tenderness or masses, suggestive of intussusception.

Investigation and diagnosis

Hx
- A history of preceding throat infection.
- The 'tetrad' of clinical features (see *OSCE tips 2*).

Ex
- Alongside identifying the typical features, it is important to exclude features of meningism.

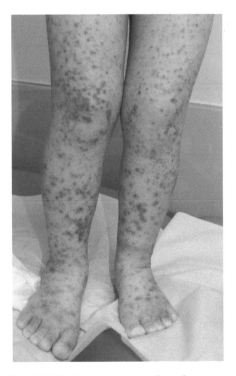

Fig. 15.20: Typical purpuric, papular rash seen in HSP.

Ix
- Diagnosis is usually clinical and based on the common tetrad; investigations are therefore to **look for renal involvement and to exclude other diagnoses**.
- Urine dipstick for blood and protein. A 24-hour urine can be tested for the volume of protein passed (>3g/day in nephrotic syndrome).
- Bloods: U&E should be performed if renal involvement is suspected. To exclude coagulopathies (e.g. idiopathic thrombocytopenic purpura (ITP) as an aetiology for the purpuric rash, clotting may also be done.

DDx
- Meningococcal septicaemia
- Intussusception
- ITP – purpuric rash
- Systemic lupus erythematosus – arthralgia and renal involvement
- Rheumatoid arthritis
- Glomerulonephritis
- Physical abuse

Management

- **Supportive and symptomatic treatment** is the mainstay of patient management, as HSP is usually self-limiting.
- Simple analgesia can be used to manage abdominal or joint pain. Care should be taken with NSAIDs in those with renal involvement.
- Where there is renal involvement, **corticosteroids** are the usual therapeutic agent but, in the presence of a rapidly progressing glomerulonephritis, immunosuppressants may be added.
- *Prognosis is generally excellent* and less than 1% of patients develop end-stage renal failure.

15.5.3 Kawasaki disease

Kawasaki disease (KD) is a **small/medium-sized vessel systemic vasculitis** that, alongside other features, presents with dermatological changes. The pathophysiology of this condition is not well understood. Rare before 6 months and after 5 years of age, it predominantly affects **north-east Asians** (particularly the Japanese), with a slight preponderance in males (1.5:1).

Clinical features

The child always has a fever (≥5/7 duration) and is highly irritable with it. The other clinical features can be found in *Fig. 15.21*. The main clinical concern is that these patients can develop coronary artery aneurysm (→ acute myocardial events) if not diagnosed and treated promptly. Untreated, ~25% of patients will develop this complication and it is the main cause of morbidity and mortality in KD.

Rapid diagnosis – Kawasaki disease

A persistent fever lasting ≥5/7 alongside ≥4 of the following:

- Widespread **polymorphic rash** – usual onset day 3–5. Starts in the peripheries and perineum before migrating to the trunk. Never vesicular.
- **Changes in the extremities** – initially, oedema and erythema of the hands and feet, later followed by desquamation of the fingers, toes and perineum.
- **Changes in the lips and oral cavity** – erythematous, cracked lips with an inflamed, red tongue ('strawberry tongue') and mucosal injection.
- Non-exudative bilateral **conjunctivitis**.
- (Unilateral) cervical **lymphadenopathy**.

Investigation and diagnosis

- There are **no diagnostic tests** for KD.
- Bloods may show ↑ CRP & ESR, ↑ Plt, ↑ ALT and bilirubin.
- Perform an **ECG** to look for conduction defects (due to myo- or pericarditis).
- An **echocardiogram** is required to look for coronary artery aneurysm.

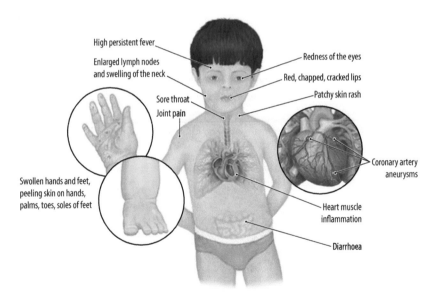

Fig. 15.21: Clinical features of Kawasaki disease.

Management

IV immunoglobulin
• Mainstay of treatment as, when given within the first 10 days of symptom onset, it significantly reduces the incidence of coronary artery aneurysm

Aspirin
• Used for its anti-inflammatory effects early in the disease process, and continued at lower dose for ~6–8/52 for its anti-platelet effects

Miscellaneous
• Admit the child • Serial echocardiograms to look for cardiac sequelae

15.5.4   Urticaria

In broad terms, urticaria is thought to be due to mast cell degranulation, releasing histamine (alongside other inflammatory mediators) into the dermis. This induces the Triple Response of Lewis: pruritus, vasodilatation ($\rightarrow$ erythema) and increased vasopermeability ($\rightarrow$ swelling/ wheal), giving rise to its classical clinical features. The aetiologies can be broadly categorized into three groups (see *Table 15.4*).

Epidemiology: affects up to one quarter of all children, with a higher incidence in those with a **history of atopy**.

Distribution: can range from a generalized distribution to a specific location, depending on the aetiology.

Appearance: intensely **pruritic 'wheals'**: these are irregular-shaped, variably sized, papular lesions with central pallor and an erythematous periphery (*Fig. 15.22*). If multiple, they can coalesce to form large erythematous patches. Lesions last from minutes to hours, but tend to have resolved entirely within a day.

Management:
- Avoidance of the causal agent.
- Non-sedating H1-receptor antihistamine (such as cetirizine or loratadine).
- If it is causing distress at night, a sedating antihistamine may be useful (chlorphenamine).

Table 15.4: Common aetiologies of acute urticarial reactions

Mechanism	Aetiology	Description
Idiopathic	n/a	In up to 50% of cases, no causal agent can be identified
Immune	Food	Should be considered in all children with an urticarial rash – the main culprits are nuts, eggs and shellfish
	Medications	Most drugs can cause a dermatological reaction, so consider this when there is a clear temporal relationship between the two
	Bites/stings	n/a
	Contact	A reaction to chemical irritants, often from a patient's workplace
	Angio-oedema	See *OSCE tips 3*
Non-immune	Physical	Caused by an array of different stimuli: cholinergic – heat, exercise and sweating; cold; sunlight exposure
	Dermatographism	Firm stroking of the skin produces an urticarial response and allows the patient to 'write' on their skin
	Opiates	Cause histamine release directly
	NSAIDs	Due to inhibition of COX-1 enzyme

OSCE tips 3: Angio-oedema

Angio-oedema has a similar pathophysiology to urticaria; however, it affects the skin layers deep to the dermis. This can lead to **swelling of the soft tissues of the larynx, oropharynx, mouth and peri-orbital region** – it is the former two that are of *immediate concern* as they can lead to **rapid compromise of the airway**.

It is associated with urticaria in ~40% of cases and, in a small number of cases, is due to a deficiency of C1-esterase inhibitor (termed **'hereditary angio-oedema'** – this causes recurrent episodes of angio-oedema throughout life).

Treatment is not always needed unless there is involvement of the airway, in which case it is treated as anaphylaxis – with **adrenaline, antihistamine and steroid**.

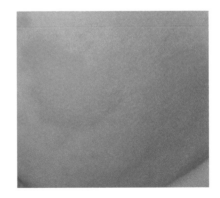

Fig. 15.22: Pruritic wheals in hives.

Chapter 16

Behavioural and genetic disorders

Autism

A spectrum of conditions ('autistic spectrum disorder'; ASD), which affect **social and communication skills** (*Fig. 16.1*).

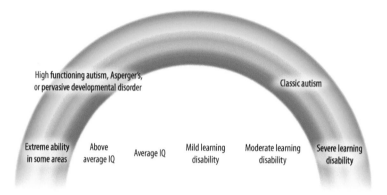

Fig. 16.1: A schematic of the autistic spectrum, from high functioning to significant disability.

Pathophysiology

- Exact mechanism not understood, appears to be multifactorial with likely genetic component.
- **Not related to parenting style or vaccinations.**

Epidemiology and risk factors

- Prevalence of **1.1% in the UK** (2011). Typically diagnosed between age 2 and 4, when children start to fall behind their peers in social and language development.
- Prevalence equal in all ethnic groups.
- **Male preponderance (5:1).**

Table 16.1: Risk factors for autistic spectrum disorder	
Male sex	• One of the most significant risk factors
Family history/other siblings affected	• There is increasing evidence of a genetic basis for ASD • Specific genetic changes have been implicated but this does not explain the broad range of presentations, which fits with multifactorial process
Fragile X syndrome	• Well-recognized association

Clinical features

ASD is characterized by the presence of **three core features**, <u>all</u> of which must be present for diagnosis: poor social skills, impaired language and repetitive behaviours. These impairments manifest clinically, as described below:

Social skills	• Poor eye contact, difficulty empathizing, social cues being missed, lack of imaginative play

Language	• Speech delay, literal interpretation of language, restricted gestures and facial expression, echolalia

Repetitive behaviour	• Hand flapping, tiptoe gait, unusual interests, strict routine adherence

A well-known variant of ASD at the lesser end of the spectrum is **Asperger's syndrome**. These children have difficulty reading social cues, have narrow interests and find social interaction challenging; however, **their language and IQ is usually normal**.

Meanwhile, at the severe end of the spectrum, children may never develop speech and may display very ritualistic behaviour.

Investigation and diagnosis

Hx
- Parents, carers or teachers may raise concern about social **behaviour**.
- More severe forms tend to present **age 2–4**, with **speech delay** and significant social impairment.
- Ask about social milestones – when did they first smile? Have they ever played with other children? Typically **development is grossly normal for the first year of life, after which there may be delay**.
- Ask about **family history**.

Establish if there is **regression** of previously acquired skills – this is only reported in a small subset of children with ASD.

Ex
- **Developmental assessment.**
- Neurological exam.
- Examine for dysmorphic features that may suggest a concomitant diagnosis.

Ix
- **Hearing test** (children with hearing impairment often have behavioural issues due to this).
- Genetic tests for fragile X and tuberous sclerosis.
- Exclusion of **metabolic conditions** such as phenylketonuria (usually excluded in infancy with **heel prick**).
- Diagnosis is made via observation of the child against **set criteria**, once other causes of delay have been excluded.

DDx
- Fragile X, tuberous sclerosis, hearing impairment, phenylketonuria, global developmental delay (for any reason)
- Normal child! Remember social and language skills are on a spectrum

Management

Management is symptomatic and holistic.

Table 16.2: Recommended management of autism

Biological	<ul><li>Management of co-morbidities such as seizure disorders (see *OSCE tips 1*)</li><li>Care should be coordinated by a community paediatrician</li><li>Antipsychotics such as risperidone are used for aggression, especially if the child injures themselves (head banging and self-mutilation are not uncommon, especially when the child becomes frustrated)</li><li>Melatonin can be used for severe sleep dysregulation</li></ul>
Psychological	<ul><li>Support groups and counselling should be encouraged for the family</li><li>Psychological co-morbidities are very common and should be managed by experienced professionals</li></ul>
Social	<ul><li>Applied Behavioural Analysis is useful for working on reducing repetitive behaviours and teaching social skills</li><li>Educational support at school</li><li>Speech and occupational therapist input</li></ul>

OSCE tips 1: Co-morbidities in autistic spectrum disorders

- Alongside the three core features of ASD, children are more likely than the general population to be affected by mental health issues and seizure disorders.
- 1 in 4 children with autism will develop seizures in early childhood or adolescence.
- 3 in 4 will have a moderate–severe learning difficulty.
- A significant number have attention issues with hyperactivity (see *Section 16.2*).

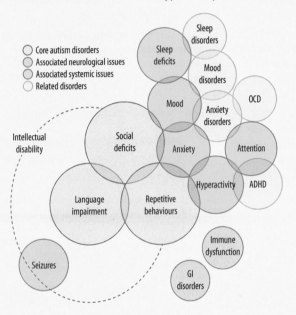

Fig. 16.2: Health issues associated with ASD.

Attention deficit hyperactivity disorder (ADHD)

ADHD is defined by the presence of **all three** of the following: hyperactivity, impulsiveness and inattention beyond what is appropriate for the child's age.

Pathophysiology

- Unclear and **multifactorial**. From twin studies → **genetic component** that seems to be related to dopaminergic and noradrenergic neural pathways.

Epidemiology and risk factors

- Prevalence depends on the specific set of diagnostic criteria that is used but is typically quoted at **2–4% of school-age children**.
- Male preponderance (4:1).

Clinical features

Symptoms

- Inattention
- Hyperactivity
- Impulsiveness

Table 16.3: Risk factors for ADHD	
Strong	Male sex
Moderate	Family history of ADHD, learning difficulties or substance misuse
Weak	*In utero* exposure to alcohol/nicotine Neurological co-morbidity

Signs

- Concerns raised by school staff or parents
- Difficulty with schooling or school refusal

Investigation and diagnosis

Rapid diagnosis – ADHD

These symptoms must persist for **more than 6 months**, in **more than one setting** and **impair** the child's social **functioning**.

Hx
- Ask about **birth**, **prenatal** history and **family history**.
- **Impulsiveness** (interrupting, difficulty taking turns).
- **Hyperactivity** (restless, fidgety, often talks excessively).
- **Inattention** (difficulty completing tasks, poor organization, lack of interest in details).

Ex
- Thorough developmental assessment and neurological examination.
- Must establish if there is **global developmental delay** or a **learning difficulty**; are there any **dysmorphic** features?
- Have **visual acuity** and **hearing** been tested?
- Observation of the parent–child relationship is also imperative.

Ix
- Diagnosis is by assessment of the child in **more than one place** (school/home) against set **diagnostic criteria**.
- Other investigations would only be done to rule out other diagnoses.

DDx
- Normal child
- Developmental delay
- Learning difficulty
- Psychological distress (bullying, abuse)
- Oppositional defiance disorder
- Seizure disorder
- Lead poisoning
- Fragile X

Management

- Half of children diagnosed with ADHD will have symptoms into adolescence and adulthood. There is a **significant association with substance abuse, risk-taking behaviour and criminality in later life**.
- Half will develop a psychiatric illness as they get older.
- Management is **multidisciplinary** and starts with **behaviour management** centred around boundaries, routine and consistency; **positive reinforcement** gives far better outcomes than the inverse. **Parental training** and **education** improve outcomes.
- **Medical management** is with stimulant medication, typically methylphenidate in the UK (see below).

Clinical pharmacology – Methylphenidate in ADHD management

- A CNS stimulant
- Its use is not advised unless non-pharmacological treatment strategies have failed
- Side-effects include anxiety, tremors, hypertension, insomnia, anorexia and hyperhidrosis, and children and families should be counselled by an experienced paediatrician prior to commencing treatment.
- Once on treatment, blood pressure must be checked annually and treatment ceased if hypertension develops

Blocks both the dopamine (DAT) and noradrenaline (NET) transporters on the synaptic membrane

↓

Inhibits the reuptake of dopamine (DA) and noradrenaline (NA)

↓

Net increase in DA and NA in **neuronal synapses**

↓

Increased neurotransmission of these substances

Down syndrome

Down syndrome is also known as trisomy 21, the most common disorder of chromosome number (aneuploidy).

Pathophysiology

- Most cases are due to **non-disjunction** of the 21st chromosome (*Fig. 16.3*). Some are due to **translocations** and an even smaller number of cases are due to **genetic mosaicism** (some cells have two and some three copies of the 21st chromosome).
- Trisomy 21 is more common because the 21st chromosome holds the smallest amount of genetic material → foetuses with an extra 21st chromosome are more likely to survive (than other trisomies).

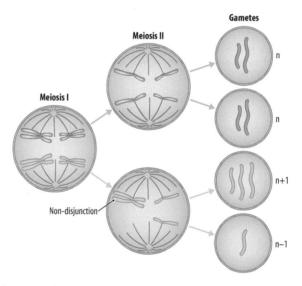

Fig. 16.3: Non-disjunction during meiosis, resulting in aneuploidy of a chromosome.

Epidemiology and risk factors

- 1:650 live births (all maternal ages)
- Prevalence increases with maternal age → 1:37 if mother >44 years old.

Table 16.4: Risk factors for Down syndrome

Strong	Increasing maternal age
Moderate	Chromosome 21 translocation in either parent
Weak	Family history

Investigation and diagnosis

Hx	
	• **Often diagnosed prenatally**.
	• If not, infant born hypotonic and often feeds poorly.
	• Other anomalies may have been identified on antenatal scans – ask!

Ex	
	• Very typical and well-recognized phenotype – see *Fig. 16.4*.
	• Note, there are many features (which are often asked in exams)

Ix • Triple testing (see *Rapid diagnosis* box). Amniocentesis. Chorionic villus sampling (offered to all women at high risk of carrying a child with Down syndrome).
• Genetic testing with a **karyotype study** usually confirms diagnosis.

DDx • Other syndromes causing dysmorphic features

OSCE tips 2: Assessing a child with Down syndrome

1. Comment on **birth history** and **how diagnosis was made**.
2. Remember there are separate **growth charts** for children with Down syndrome as they are constitutionally smaller than other children.
3. Look for **scars** indicating previous **surgery** (chest for cardiac repairs, abdomen for GI repairs or current/previous gastrostomies).

Clinical features

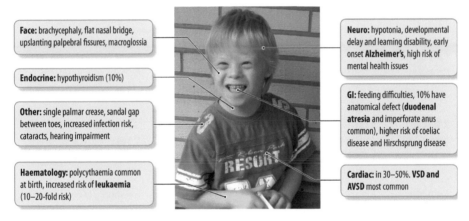

Face: brachycephaly, flat nasal bridge, upslanting palpebral fissures, macroglossia

Endocrine: hypothyroidism (10%)

Other: single palmar crease, sandal gap between toes, increased infection risk, cataracts, hearing impairment

Haematology: polycythaemia common at birth, increased risk of **leukaemia** (10–20-fold risk)

Neuro: hypotonia, developmental delay and learning disability, early onset **Alzheimer's**, high risk of mental health issues

GI: feeding difficulties, 10% have anatomical defect (**duodenal atresia** and imperforate anus common), higher risk of coeliac disease and Hirschsprung disease

Cardiac: in 30–50%. **VSD and AVSD** most common

Fig. 16.4: Clinical features of Down syndrome.

Management

• Differs depending on each child's specific needs.
• A large proportion will have a congenital anomaly requiring surgery, often very early in life.
• Feeding issues are common secondary to hypotonia → babies may need NG feeding support.
• A child with Down syndrome and their family will need ongoing medical, social and psychological support throughout the child's life.

Rapid diagnosis – triple testing

This is a prenatal maternal test which looks at three markers:
• alpha-fetoprotein (AFP)
• human chorionic gonadotrophin (hCG)
• Unconjugated oestradiol (UE$_3$)

The results are used to classify if the pregnancy is high- or low-risk for Down syndrome (**high risk = ↓AFP, ↑hCG, ↓UE$_3$**)

16.4 Genetic syndromes

There are a vast number of genetic syndromes; here, we cover some of the common conditions that you should be aware of and which often come up in medical school exams.

16.4.1 Mendelian inheritance

Pathophysiology

It is important you understand modes of inheritance **so you can counsel families on future risk** and ascertain a mode of inheritance from a careful family history and family tree (*Table 16.5*).

Table 16.5: Patterns of inheritance

Pattern	Inheritance	Examples
Autosomal dominant	50% chance of inheritance if one parent has condition.	Achondroplasia, neurofibromatosis, Marfan's, Huntington's
Autosomal recessive	If both parents are carriers, the child has a (i) 25% chance of having the condition; (ii) 50% chance of being a carrier themselves; (iii) 25% chance of being an unaffected non-carrier.	Cystic fibrosis, sickle cell disease, phenylketonuria
X-linked dominant	If **father** affected – daughter always affected, son never. If **mother** affected – daughter 50% affected, son 50% affected.	X-linked vitamin D-resistant rickets, Rett syndrome, fragile X syndrome
X-linked recessive	Almost exclusively affects males. (i) If mother is a carrier – 50% chance daughter is a carrier, 50% chance son affected by condition; (ii) if father affected – 100% daughters carriers, 0% sons affected.	Haemophilia A, Duchenne muscular dystrophy, G6PD, colour blindness
Uniparental disomy	Both copies of a chromosome are inherited from one parent. Karyotype is normal.	Prader–Willi syndrome, Angelman syndrome

Epidemiology and risk factors

- Chromosomal abnormalities are present in 0.5% of live births.
- 30–50% of paediatric inpatients have a congenital malformation or genetic syndrome.

Investigation and diagnosis

Ix
- **Karyotype** – visualizes chromosomes, showing abnormalities in structure and number.
- **FISH (fluorescent *in situ* hybridization)** – looks for specific sequences on chromosomes: are there too many or not enough?
- **Microarray comparative genomic hybridization** – looks for chromosomal imbalances and can look at more material than FISH.

16.4.2 Chromosomal abnormalities

Clinical features

Non-Mendelian inherited disorders are typically due to chromosomal abnormalities that develop *in utero*. 1 in 25 oocytes and 1 in 10 spermatozoa have a chromosomal abnormality present, a **large number of which result in early miscarriage before 12 weeks' gestation**. Those that survive tend to have complex multisystem sequelae. There may be an abnormal number of chromosomes (**aneuploidy**) or deletion of part of a chromosome. The most common is trisomy 21 (Down syndrome – see *Section 16.3*).

Condition	Genetics/ incidence	Typical features
Edwards syndrome	Trisomy 18. 1:8000	Small, micrognathia, prominent occiput, cleft lip/palate, cardiac defects, overlapping fingers, 'rocker bottom' feet, severe developmental delay. >**90% don't survive to 1 year**.
Patau syndrome	Trisomy 13. 1:14 000	Microcephaly, small eyes, scalp defects, cleft lip/palate, cardiac defects, renal abnormalities, polydactyly, severe developmental delay. >**90% don't survive to 6 months**.
Turner syndrome	45,X. 1:2500 females	Infertility, short stature, primary amenorrhoea, pubertal delay, **webbed neck**, low-set ears, normal intelligence, wide-spaced nipples, horseshoe kidney (50%), cardiac defects (especially coarctation of the aorta).
Klinefelter syndrome	47,XXY. 1:1000 males	**Hypogonadism**, infertility, **tall**, long limbs, gynaecomastia in adolescence.
Williams syndrome	7q11.2 deletion	**Elfin facies**, blue stellate irises, moderate intellectual impairment but often strong social skills with so-called '**cocktail party personality**'. 80% have cardiac defect, usually aortic or pulmonary stenosis.

(continued)

Condition	Genetics/ incidence	Typical features
DiGeorge syndrome	22q11.2 deletion	Damage to 3rd and 4th pharyngeal arches *in utero*. Often referred to as '**CATCH-22**': **C**ardiac anomalies **A**bnormal facies **T**hymic hypoplasia **C**left palate **H**ypocalcaemia **22**q11.2 deletion

Management

- **Multidisciplinary** team management, often under tertiary paediatric care teams.
- **Genetic counselling** for families around risk to further children/whether affected child will be able to have children.
- **Psychological support** for families and good relationships with paediatric teams essential. Many of these children will have short life expectancy and not be able to be independent as they grow up; will need long-term support.

Appendix A

System-specific symptoms

Here we list some of the most common symptoms from each major system of the body and, where possible, correlate them with the anatomical location or pathological process that they are most closely related to.

Due to the subtleties of medicine, these lists are crude, inexact and abbreviated. They are only intended to provide the reader with a basic framework upon which to base their history taking, the art of which can only be learnt experientially through clinical teaching and practice.

Cardiovascular system

Cardiac failure

Poor feeding
Pedal swelling
Breathlessness with feeding

Valvular disease

Syncope/pre-syncope, often associated with activity

Arrhythmia

Palpitations
Syncope / pre-syncope, unrelated to activity

Non-specific

Chest pain / tightness / heaviness
Breathlessness (if exertional – consider cardiac failure or valvular disease; if unrelated to activity – consider arrhythmia)

Dermatological system

Symptoms of the lesion(s)

Itchy?
Painful?
Discharge and/or bleeding?

Appearance of the lesion

Colour?
Size?
Initial distribution and spread over time?
Intermittent or constant?

Gastrointestinal tract

Oesophagus

Odynophagia
Dysphagia

Stomach

Dyspepsia

Small bowel

Nil specific

Large bowel

Nil specific

Rectum

Faecal urgency
Abdominal pain relieved by defecation

Hepatobiliary and pancreas

RUQ pain
Jaundice (if obstructive, pale stools and dark urine accompany this)
Steatorrhoea

Non-specific

Nausea and vomiting
Haematemesis
Abdominal pain (epigastrium – foregut, periumbilical – midgut, suprapubic – hindgut)
Abdominal distension
Weight loss

Diarrhoea
Constipation
Flatus
Per rectum (PR) bleeding

Genitourinary tract

Kidneys and ureter

Loin and/or groin pain

Bladder

Dysuria
Urgency
Frequency
Incomplete voiding

Prostate and urethra

Hesitancy
Straining
Poor stream
Terminal dribbling

Non-specific

Haematuria
Abdominal pain
Nocturia

Musculoskeletal system

Non-specific

Pain
Stiffness
Swelling
Erythema
Clicking
Locking
Deformity

Following trauma

Distal sensory deficit
Distal motor deficit
Pain elsewhere

In inflammatory arthropathies

Which joint affected first?
The progression of the joints affected? Is it symmetrical or asymmetrical?
When is stiffness worse? (tends to be worse in the morning and improve with the day)
How long does stiffness last?
A full systemic enquiry is also important.

Nervous system

Positive neurology

Stiffness / rigidity
Unintended movements
Sensory changes (e.g. pain)

Negative neurology

Weakness
Sensory changes (e.g. paraesthesia or numbness)

Cranial nerves

I (Olfactory) – change in sense of smell
II (Optic) – reduced visual acuity
III (Oculomotor) – diplopia
IV (Trochlear) – diplopia
V (Trigeminal) – sensory changes on the face / deviation of mandible towards affected side
VI (Abducens) – diplopia
VII (Facial) – facial paralysis / ptosis
VIII (Vestibulocochlear) – sensorineural hearing loss / vertigo
IX (Glossopharyngeal) – dysphagia (mild) / palatal and pharyngeal sensory loss
X (Vagus) – dysphagia / hoarseness
XI (Accessory) – weakness of head turning (sternocleidomastoid) / weakness of shoulder shrug (trapezius)
XII (Hypoglossal) – atrophy of the tongue

Cerebellum

Incoordination
Dysarthria
Ataxia
Dysphagia

Respiratory system

Upper respiratory tract

Sore throat
Hoarseness
Stridor
Dribbling
Cervical lymphadenopathy

Lower respiratory tract

Chest pain
Wheeze

Non-specific

Breathlessness
Cough
Haemoptysis

Appendix B

Image acknowledgements

Fig. 1.1
Adapted from image at www.thefreedictionary.com

Fig. 1.2
Reproduced from Pikala,T.R. *et al.*, Wilson's disease with a rare presentation: resistant rickets, *Indian Journal of Health Sciences and Biomedical Research* (2015) with permission from Wolters Kluwer Medknow Publications

Fig. 1.3
Reproduced under a Creative Commons Attribution-Share Alike 3.0 Unported Licence. Available at https://commons.wikimedia.org/wiki/File:Hernie_ligne_blanche.JPG

Fig. 1.5
Reproduced from http://casemed.case.edu/clerkships/neurology/NeurLrngObjectives/Floppy%20Baby.htm

Fig. 1.6
Adapted from image at www.thefreedictionary.com

Fig. 3.2
Reproduced from https://factrepublic.com/facts/2728/

Unnumbered image of newborn in *Section 3.2* reproduced under licence from stock.adobe.com

Fig. 3.3
Reproduced from Meeks, M., Hallsworth, M. and Yeo, H. *Nursing the Neonate*, 2nd edition, with permission from Wiley-Blackwell

Fig. 3.5
Reproduced with permission from www.learningradiology.com

Fig. 3.6
Adapted from image at www.omicsonline.org

Fig. 3.7
Reproduced with permission from www.med-ed.virginia.edu/courses/rad/peds/neuro_webpages/b19.html

Fig. 3.8
Reproduced with permission from www.learningradiology.com

Fig. 3.9
Reproduced from www.adhb.govt.nz/newborn/Guidelines/Developmental/ROP.htm

Fig. 3.10
Adapted from image at http://priscillacyun.wixsite.com/

Fig. 3.11
Adapted from image at https://microbiologyinfo.com

Fig. 3.12

Adapted from image in NICE (2010) CG98, *Jaundice in Newborn Babies under 28 Days*

Fig. 3.13

Reproduced from *Mayo Clin Proc*, 73(1), Lefkowitch, J.H., Biliary atresia, 90–5, 1998, with permission from Elsevier

Fig. 3.14

Adapted from image at www.mountnittany.org

Fig. 3.15

Republished with permission of Vinod K. Bhutani, from *Care of the Jaundiced Neonate*, Stevenson, D.K., Maisels, M.J. and Watchko, J.F., 2012; permission conveyed through Copyright Clearance Center, Inc.

Fig. 3.16

Reproduced from Central Lakes Medical (www.centrallakesclinic.biz) under a Creative Commons Attribution 3.0 Licence

Fig. 3.17

Adapted from image at https://nursingcrib.com

Fig. 3.18

Reproduced from *Cleft Lip and Palate Surgery*, by Koroush Taheri Talesh and Mohammed Hosein Kalantar Motamedi (www.intechopen.com/books/a-textbook-of-advanced-oral-and-maxillofacial-surgery/cleft-lip-and-palate-surgery) under a Creative Commons Attribution 3.0 Licence

Figs. 3.19 and 4.1

Adapted from image by Centers for Disease Control and Prevention

Fig. 4.2

Reproduced from http://diaperbagconfessions.com

Fig. 5.1

Reproduced from *Archives of Disease in Childhood: Education & Practice*, Maguire, S., Which injuries may indicate child abuse? 95(6): 170–7, 2010, with permission from BMJ Publishing Group Ltd

Figs. 5.2 and 5.4a

Adapted from *Pediatric Clinics*, 37, Johnson, C.F., Inflicted injury versus accidental injury (1990), with permission from Elsevier

Fig. 5.4b

Reproduced from www.abusewatch.net

Fig. 5.5a

Reproduced from *Archives of Disease in Childhood*, Hobbs, C.J., When are burns not accidental? **61** (4), 1986, with permission from BMJ Publishing Group Ltd.

Fig. 5.5b

Reproduced from http://clinicalgate.com

Fig. 5.6

Reproduced from www.abusewatch.net

Fig. 5.7

Image courtesy of Jonathan Thackeray, MD, Dayton Children's Hospital

Fig. 6.2

© NICE (2013) Feverish illness in children, CG160. Available from www.nice.org.uk/guidance/cg160 All rights reserved. Subject to Notice of rights. NICE guidance is prepared for the National Health Service in England. All NICE guidance is subject to regular review and may be updated or withdrawn. NICE accepts no responsibility for the use of its content in this product/publication.

Fig. 7.1

Adapted with permission from image at https://library.med.utah.edu

Fig. 7.2

Adapted from image at 1sc.in/blood-allergy-test

Fig. 8.1

Reproduced under a CC BY 3.0 licence. Attribution: Blausen.com staff (2014) "Medical gallery of Blausen Medical 2014". *WikiJournal of Medicine* **1** (2). DOI:10.15347/wjm/2014.010. ISSN 2002–4436. Own work.

Fig. 8.2

Reproduced with permission from www.hearourheart.org

Fig. 8.3

Reproduced from www.medrevise.co.uk

Fig. 8.4

Reproduced from www.slideshare.net

Fig. 8.5

Adapted from image at www.nationwidechildrens.org

Fig. 8.6

Reproduced from www.med-ed.virginia.edu

Fig. 8.8

Reproduced under a Creative Commons Attribution non-Commercial Share-Alike 3.0 Licence. Available at http://www.wikiradiography.net/page/Chest+Radiography+for+Inhaled+Foreign+Body

Fig. 8.9

Reproduced from https://hubpages.com/health

Fig. 8.10

Adapted from image at http://sphweb.bumc.bu.edu

Fig. 8.12

Adapted from image at stock.adobe.com

Fig. 9.2

Adapted from image at http://staticl.squarespace.com

Fig. 9.4

Reproduced from www.natural-health-news.com

Fig. 9.5

Reproduced with permission from Medscape Drugs & Diseases (https://emedicine.medscape.com/), Hirschsprung Disease Imaging, 2015, available at https://emedicine.medscape.com/article/409150-overview

Fig. 9.6

Adapted from image at www.heartlandqc.com

Fig. 9.8

Reproduced from Hatfield, N.T. and Kincheloe, C., *Introductory Maternity and Pediatric Nursing*, 2017, with permission from Wolters Kluwer.

Fig. 9.9

Reproduced with permission from DermNetNZ

Fig. 9.10

Adapted from image at www.stanfordchildrens.org

Fig. 9.11

Reproduced from tdmu.edu.ua

Fig. 9.12

Adapted from image at https://commons.wikivet.net

Fig. 9.14

Reproduced with permission from Dr Taco Geertsma at www.ultrasoundcases.info

Fig. 9.15

Reproduced with permission from Loren Yamamoto, MD, MPH

Fig. 9.16

Reproduced with permission from Medscape Drugs & Diseases (https://emedicine. medscape.com/), Meckel Diverticulum Imaging, 2015, available at: https://emedicine. medscape.com/article/410644-overview

Fig. 10.1

Adapted from image at https://en.wikipedia.org/wiki/Ventricular_septal_defect#/media/ File:Vsd_simple-lg.jpg

Fig. 10.2

Adapted from image at https://radiologykey.com

Fig. 10.4

Reproduced with permission from Baylor College of Medicine

Fig. 10.5

Adapted from image at www.stanfordchildrens.org

Fig. 10.6

Reproduced with permission from P.S. Rao

Fig. 10.7

Reproduced from https://biology-forums.com

Fig. 10.8

Reproduced with permission from Holt International.

Fig. 10.9

Adapted from image at www.stanfordchildrens.org

Fig. 10.10

Adapted from image at www.kidsheartshouston.com

Fig. 10.11

Reproduced from www.newmedicalterms.com

Fig. 10.12

Adapted from image at https://connect.mayoclinic.org

Fig. 10.13

Reproduced under a Creative Commons Attribution-Share Alike 3.0 Unported Licence. Available at: https://en.wikipedia.org/wiki/Tricuspid_atresia#/media/File:Tricuspid_atresia.svg Additional attribution RupertMillard

Fig. 10.15

By James Heilman, MD – Own work, CC BY-SA 3.0, https://commons.wikimedia.org/w/index.php?curid=24076834

Fig. 10.16

Reproduced from https://lifeinthefastlane.com

Fig. 10.17

Reproduced from https://smartypance.com

Fig. 11.1

Reproduced from https://syndromepictures.com

Fig. 11.2

Reproduced from http://pendidikanpesakit.myhealth.gov.my/en/2001/

Fig. 11.3

Adapted from image at www.sterlingcare.com

Fig. 11.4

Reproduced from http://body-disease.com

Fig. 11.7

Reproduced under a Creative Commons CC0 1.0 Universal Public Domain Dedication. Available at: https://commons.wikimedia.org/wiki/File:Hypospadias-lg.jpg

Fig. 11.8

Adapted from image from EAU Patient Information, patients.uroweb.org

Fig. 12.1

Reproduced from http://www.oncetus.com/sozluk/brudzinski_bulgusu/

Fig. 12.3

Reproduced from https://pedclerk.bsd.uchicago.edu/page/breath-holding-spells

Fig. 12.5

Reproduced from *Journal of Pediatric Neurosciences*, Venkataramana, N.K., Spinal dysraphism, 2011, 6(3): 31–40, with permission from Wolters Kluwer Medknow Publications

Fig. 12.6

Adapted from image at www.tri-stateneurosurgery.com

Fig. 12.8a

Reproduced courtesy of RegionalDerm.com

Fig. 12.8b

Reproduced with permission from www.mrcophth.com/

Fig. 12.8c

Reproduced from www.gudhealth.com

Fig. 12.8d

Reproduced under a Creative Commons Attribution 4.0 International Licence. Available at: https://en.wikipedia.org/wiki/Lisch_nodule#/media/File:Lisch_nodules.jpg. Author: Dimitrios Malamos

Fig. 12.9

Reproduced from *EMBO Molecular Medicine*, Neuman, N.A. and Henske, E.P., Non-canonical functions of the tuberous sclerosis complex-Rheb signalling axis, 2011, **3** (4): 12, with permission from John Wiley and Sons

Fig. 12.10a and b

Reproduced with permission from DermNetNZ

Fig. 12.11

Adapted from image at https://rehabathome.tumblr.com/image/157870878914

Fig. 13.1

Reproduced with permission from Radiologypics.com; contributor Jeffrey L. Koning, MD.

Figs. 13.2 and 13.3

Reproduced with permission from www.radiologyassistant.nl

Fig. 13.4

Reproduced with permission from Diagnostic Imaging Pathways (http://www.imagingpathways.health.wa.gov.au)

Fig. 13.6

Reproduced under a Creative Commons Attribution-Share Alike 3.0 Unported licence. Available at: https://commons.wikimedia.org/wiki/File:Scoliosis_Cobb.jpg. Attribution: Skoliose-Info-Forum.de

Fig. 13.7

Adapted from image at https://rad.washington.edu

Fig. 13.8

Reproduced under a Creative Commons Attribution-Share Alike 4.0 International Licence. Available at: https://upload.wikimedia.org/wikipedia/commons/0/0b/ScheuermannDiseaseT6to10.png. Author: James Heilman, MD.

Fig. 13.9

Reproduced under a Creative Commons Attribution 4.0 International Licence. Attribution: (2015). "THE SEVERAL FACES OF SCHMORL'S NODE: PICTORIAL ESSAY". *Coluna/Columna* **14** (4): 320–323.

Fig. 13.10a

Reproduced from https://clinicalgate.com

Fig. 13.10b

Reproduced from www.slideshare.net/z2jeetendra/nail-changes-on-different-dermatologic-disease

Fig. 13.11a

Reproduced from www.oocities.org/thetolesle/

Fig. 13.11b

Reproduced from www.yabibo.com

Fig. 13.12a
Reproduced with permission from Medscape Drugs & Diseases (https://emedicine.medscape.com/), Juvenile Dermatomyositis, 2016, available at: https://emedicine.medscape.com/article/1417215-overview

Fig. 13.12b
Reproduced under a Creative Commons Attribution-Share Alike 3.0 Unported licence. Available at: https://commons.wikimedia.org/wiki/File:Dermatomyositis2.jpg. Authors: Elizabeth M. Dugan, Adam M. Huber, Frederick W. Miller & Lisa G. Rider

Fig. 13.13
Adapted from image at advanceweb.com

Fig. 13.14
Reproduced under a Creative Commons Attribution-Share Alike 1.0 Generic licence. Available at: https://en.wikipedia.org/wiki/Rickets#/media/File:XrayRicketsLegssmall.jpg. Additional attribution: Mrich.
Unnumbered images in Section 13.6.1: reproduced from https://image.slidesharecdn.com

Fig. 13.15
Reproduced with permission.

Fig. 14.1
Reproduced with permission from https://library.med.utah.edu

Figs. 14.2 and 14.5
Reproduced from www.memorangapp.com

Fig. 14.4
Reproduced from http://media.mssm.edu/blood/morphology_tutorial_scigliano/4677.html

Fig. 14.6
Reproduced from https://pedclerk.bsd.uchicago.edu

Fig. 14.7
Adapted from image at www.stepwards.com

Fig. 14.8
Reproduced from Lobet, S., Hermans, C, and Lambert, C., Optimal management of hemophilic arthropathy and hematomas, *Journal of Blood Medicine*, 2014, 5: 207–18, with permission from Dr Sébastien Lobet

Fig. 14.9
Adapted from image at https://haemophilia.ie

Fig. 14.10
Reproduced from www.tabletsmanual.com

Figs. 15.1–15.7, 15.8b, 15.9a, 15.10a, b, 15.11a, 15.13a, b, 15.16, 15.17a, b, 15.18a, 15.19a
Reproduced with permission from DermNetNZ

Fig. 15.8a
Reproduced under a Creative Commons Attribution 2.5 Generic licence. Available at: https://en.wikipedia.org/wiki/Scarlet_fever#/media/File:Scarlet_fever_2.jpg. Attribution: Estreya

Fig. 15.8c
Reproduced under a Creative Commons Attribution-Share Alike 3.0 Unported licence.

Available at: https://en.wikipedia.org/wiki/Scarlet_fever#/media/File:Skarlatina.jpg.
Attribution: Afag Azizova

Fig. 15.9b

Reproduced from infantigoinfo.com

Fig. 15.11b

Reproduced from herd-effect.tumblr.com

Fig. 15.12

Centers for Disease Control and Prevention.

Fig. 15.14

Reproduced from *Dermatology Made Easy* by A. Oakley. Scion Publishing Ltd, 2017

Fig. 15.15a

Reproduced under a Creative Commons Attribution-Share Alike 3.0 Unported Licence.
Available at: https://en.wikipedia.org/wiki/Hand,_foot,_and_mouth_disease#/media/
File:Hand_Foot_Mouth_Disease.png. Attribution: MidgleyDJ

Fig. 15.15b

Reproduced under a Creative Commons Attribution-Share Alike 3.0 Unported Licence.
Available at: https://upload.wikimedia.org/wikipedia/commons/c/c5/Hand_foot_and_
mouth_disease_on_child_feet.jpg. Attribution: Ngufra

Fig. 15.18b

Reproduced from https://en.wikipedia.org/wiki/Scabies#/media/File:Scabies-burrow.jpg.
Attribution: Michael Geary. Public domain

Fig. 15.19b

Reproduced from www.dermexpert.co.uk

Fig. 15.19c

Reproduced under a Creative Commons Attribution 2.0 Generic licence. Available at: https://
commons.wikimedia.org/wiki/Category:Eczema#/media/File:Eczema_(14100950936).jpg.
Attribution: NIAID

Fig. 15.19d

Reproduced from www.medskin.co.uk, with permission from Dr Inma Mauri-Sole

Fig. 15.20

Reproduced from http://derminaminute.com

Fig. 15.21

Adapted from image at diseasesforum.com

Fig. 15.22

Reproduced from http://reliefforhives.blogspot.com

Fig. 16.3

Adapted from figure in *New Clinical Genetics*, 3rd edition, Read, A. and Donnai, D.
Scion Publishing Ltd, 2015

Fig. 16.4

Adapted from image on Wikipedia, reproduced under a Creative Commons Attribution-
Share Alike 3.0 Unported licence. Available at: https://en.wikipedia.org.uk/wiki/Down_
syndrome#/media/File:Boy_with_Down_syndrome.jpg. Attribution: Vanellus Foto.

Index